ENDING THE SOCIAL CARE CRISIS

A New Road to Reform

Richard Humphries

First published in Great Britain in 2022 by

Policy Press, an imprint of
Bristol University Press
University of Bristol
1-9 Old Park Hill
Bristol
BS2 8BB
UK
t: +44 (0)117 374 6645
e: bup-info@bristol.ac.uk

Details of international sales and distribution partners are available at
policy.bristoluniversitypress.co.uk

British Library Cataloguing in Publication Data
A catalogue record for this book is available from the British Library

ISBN 978-1-4473-6445-0 paperback
ISBN 978-1-4473-6446-7 ePub
ISBN 978-1-4473-6447-4 ePdf

Cover design: Liam Roberts Design
Front cover image: iStock/timsa
Bristol University Press and Policy Press use environmentally
responsible print partners.
Printed in Great Britain by CMP, Poole

For my parents

Contents

List of figures, tables and boxes

Figures

Tables

Boxes

1

Introduction

I shall be telling this with a sigh
Somewhere ages and ages hence:
Two roads diverged in a wood, and I
I took the one less travelled by,
And that has made all the difference.

Robert Frost, 'The Road Not Taken'

Promises, promises

On a sunny summer morning on the steps of 10 Downing Street in 2019, newly elected Prime Minister Boris Johnson declared that he would "fix the crisis in social care once and for all with a clear plan we have prepared to give every older person the dignity and security they deserve. My job," he said, "is to protect you or your parents or grandparents from the fear of having to sell your home to pay for the costs of care" (HM Government, 2019). It was to be over two years later before a plan, and then a very early-stage plan, was to materialise. Now rewind to 1997 and Brighton where a fresh-faced newly elected Prime Minister Tony Blair told his party conference that "I don't want [our children] brought up in a country where the only way pensioners can get long-term care is by selling their home" (Blair, 1997). It is telling that both prime ministers, separated by 22 years and big political differences, both defined the 'problem' of social care as being about older people – and, more precisely, older people having to sell their homes to pay for care. Arguably, this narrow and distorted view has unhelpfully channelled much of the political debate down a particular route. It has contributed to a legacy of neglect and indifference to what is one of the most pressing domestic policy challenges of our time.

In truth, although older people – defined in this book as aged 65 and over (though whether 65 is really that old any more is another matter) – are the biggest group of people who use council-funded social care, the number has been falling in recent years, despite our ageing population. At the same time, more working-age people, usually with disabilities or other kinds of need, are getting support. They now account for almost a half of what councils spend on social care. Currently one in three people aged between 16 and 64 in the UK has a long-term health condition, and one in five people aged between 16 and 64 in the UK has a disability. The number of working-age people reporting a disability increased by 20 per cent between 2013 and 2019, and is forecast to continue to grow (Department of Work and Pensions, 2021). This is not just about older people. Any of us, at any age, might need care and support.

Nor is it just about care homes. Most people, whatever their age, get their care and support in their own homes – which is as it should be. And most of those living in care homes do not end up selling their homes to pay for it (and arguably no one should have to because of an arrangement called a deferred payment that enables care home fees to be paid from the person's estate after their death). There are other reasons, explained later, why the issue of 'selling your home to pay for care' has generated such a huge amount of publicity and political noise out of all proportion to the relatively small numbers of people affected. So, we should not be surprised that various efforts to sort out the 'crisis' in social care have floundered when the framing of the problem to be solved has been so skewed.

Nevertheless, it has been through the lens of care homes that social care has made the news, and the experiences of the COVID-19 pandemic that have cost the lives of over 27,000 residents in England alone and doubled the risk of death for care workers – this despite protestations about the 'protective ring' the government claimed to have thrown round them. It may well be, as the House of Commons Health Select Committee concluded, that 'the toll the pandemic has taken on this sector means that social care is no longer a hidden problem, but one that the country as a whole understands' (House of Commons Health and Social Care Committee, 2021). It is certainly true that many of the problems exposed so rawly in the news bulletins and newspapers during the pandemic were there long before our lives were turned upside down. COVID-19 did not cause most of these problems but has magnified them (Dunn et al, 2021).

Social care – the price of success?

In truth, what today we call social care covers a kaleidoscope of needs and circumstances across all ages that defy individual categorisation. Its vast span can cover a 19-year-old with autism at one end of the spectrum of adulthood to a 90-year-old with dementia at the other (Chapter 3 will consider in more depth what is meant by social care and what it covers). For many of us, our needs for social care, like our needs for health care, are concentrated at the end of our lives, but they can arise at any age for any number of reasons but often involving illness, infirmity and sometimes plain ill-fortune. It could be an accident, a stroke, a fall, a descent into dependence on drugs or alcohol, a chronic health problem, an episode of mental illness, the frailty that comes with being very old, the experience or risk of abuse or exploitation. Any permutation of these and other events will leave most of us at some point of our lives needing help of some kind to lead our lives with as much independence, dignity and choice as possible. The nature of that help varies so much. It can involve needing a lot of support with personal care – 'activities of daily living' in the jargon – typically help with getting in and out of bed, getting dressed, having a shower or a bath; or it might be short-term help to get back on our feet after a spell of illness or hospitalisation. For many, it is less about a narrow range of functional care needs and more about help and support to live independently, to maintain friendships and social networks in the place we live, to hold down a job or attend college or university. Most of us will get this help in our own homes. Whatever our particular needs and circumstances, social care is the key to unlocking the possibility of living the best life we can.

The new importance of social care (described in many countries as long-term care) across the developed world is driven by the rapid march of social and economic progress over the last 150 years. Back in the 1940s when the welfare state was created, not that many people lived long enough to need care and those that did were poor enough to get it free. Mostly, this was institutional care in former workhouse buildings and long-stay hospital wards. Few people had homes to sell. Instead, universal health care was the big priority. Alongside the popular acclaim for the newly created NHS – the poster-boy of the welfare state – the opening words of the parallel legislation for 'welfare' services said it all: 'an Act to eliminate the Poor Law.' Non-medical care, or social care as it is termed today, was not an issue then. It spent the next 75 years in the shadows of its bigger and better-known sibling. The architects of the welfare state could not have imagined how much would change, not least the startling prospect that at least a third of babies born in 2019 will live to the age of 100 (Gratton and Scott, 2016). Economist and former national statistics chief Andrew Dilnot tells a story about the myth of a golden age when grandma was looked after in the bosom of her family, sitting by the inglenook fireplace knitting socks for her grandchildren. It was a myth, he explains, because grandma didn't exist – grandma was dead.

These changes have profound consequences for all of us, not just those in later life. We are living longer at all ages. Medical advances means that babies born with severe problems are surviving and children with disabilities are living well into adulthood if not old age. Social care is an all-ages issue. Improvements in public health have conquered infectious diseases, at least until COVID-19 came along. These have since been displaced by chronic long-term health problems that we will live with, not die from. They will cause us to need more health and social care in the long term. We are generally much better off and many of us enjoy wealth that puts financial help from the state out of reach – because, unlike health care, social care is not free at the point of use.

The combined effect of all these changes is that social care is now coming out of the shadows. More of us will need care and support and, under the current rules, many of us will have to pay for it ourselves. This not about some minority group apart from the rest of society, but a universal need affecting all of us – our grandparents, parents, possibly our children, our friends and neighbours, and eventually ourselves.

Falling behind

It has often been said that success has many parents but failure is always an orphan. It is striking that the crisis of social care, unlike so many challenges of our modern age, such as climate change, crime, or racial injustice, is borne of success, not failure, in the way our lives and longevity have been transformed by social and economic progress. But, instead of seeing this as a cause for celebration and facing up to the consequences for the care we need, too many policy-makers and commentators have descended into a gloomy and overwhelmingly negative language of 'demographic timebombs', the financial burden and costs of care and the threat it poses to our property wealth. Usually, this is accompanied by a political narrative that places social care in the 'too difficult' box – a toxic issue that is seen by national politicians as a threat to votes and electability.

As a result, although society has changed out of all recognition, the way social care works – how it is organised, funded and delivered – has not kept pace. For people needing care and support today, the kind of services they will be offered – essentially residential care, domiciliary (home) care and day care – has changed very little since the 1950s (NHS Digital, 2020a). That is not to say there have been no improvements in how those services are provided. Standards of care are now defined and regulated, with more emphasis on giving people choice, dignity and control – the philosophy of 'personalisation'. There is a much stronger push these days to avoid people having to move into a care home, especially when discharged from hospital. After all, most, if not all, of us would prefer to live in our own homes, as independently as possible, for as long as possible. And there have been some positive innovations through new services such as direct payments and personal budgets (which people use to shape their own support for example by employing their own personal assistants – PAs – instead of services contracted by the council); 'shared lives' schemes (involving people sharing their home with someone who needs support) and the expansion of extra-care housing schemes as alternatives to residential care. Many of these newer models of care have been successful and popular, as judged by the people who use them, but those that benefit from them remain in the minority. Despite a few interesting topological bumps, the landscape of care services has remained stubbornly resistant to change. Most people who need a great deal of care find that moving into a traditional care home is the only viable option. Within the world of social care, there has been much talk about the 'transformation' of adult social care, but the actual pace of change has been not so much transformational as geological.

It is not just that social care has lagged behind these changing times – in some important respects it has gone backwards. The contrast with the NHS could not be starker. In recent years, we have enjoyed faster access to a wider range of health care services, in no small measure due to a tripling of the NHS budget since 1997. The amount of care provided by the NHS has almost doubled in less than two decades (114 per cent between 2000–01 and 2017–18) (Tallack et al, 2020). Social care has travelled in a completely opposite direction. By 2019, adult social care spending per person, taking account of inflation, was 7.5 per cent lower than it was in 2010 (Institute of Fiscal Studies, 2021). It is now much harder to get social care support than it used to be, unless you are in a position to pay for it yourself. Fifteen years ago, most councils were providing care to those assessed as having 'moderate' needs. Now, almost all councils limit help to people with the highest needs. These developments are demography defying. Over the last decade alone, the number of older people has soared by almost 25 per cent, yet fewer people are getting help from councils (Tallack et al, 2020). The impact of COVID-19 has piled on the pressure. Although NHS waiting lists for treatment cause great political angst, less attention has been given to the 300,000 people who, by August 2021, were waiting for their care needs to be assessed or reviewed and support to be offered – a 25 per cent increase in just three months (ADASS, 2021a). The consequences of this are to put more pressure on unpaid family carers, usually women, who outnumber the paid care workforce by at least two to one.

Even if people pass the 'needs' test of local authority assessment, they have the further hurdle of the means test to surmount. This has not been uprated since 2010. Put simply, if you have more than £23,250 in savings or assets, which will usually include the value of your home, you will be expected to pay all of your care home costs yourself (Foster, 2021). This was described as social care's "nasty little secret" by former social care minister Paul Burstow at a King's Fund breakfast event in 2011 (King's Fund, 2011). But for more and more people, the secret is out. The rapid expansion of home ownership from the 1970s onwards has seen more people excluded from the council-funded system. How much you have to pay is not straightforward and might depend on where you live. The charity Independent Age produces a guide to paying for care aimed at older people – it runs to 44 pages. As we shall see, most people don't realise the extent of their liabilities for paying for care until it is too late to do anything about it.

The contrast with the NHS, which, despite current pressures, still aims to meet a wide range of health care needs and remains largely free at the point of use, has become even starker for people who have a mixture of health and care needs that are hard to disentangle. In the early days of the community care reforms in the 1990s, I recall anguished debates with health service colleagues about the differences between a 'health' bath – one provided by a district nurse, in which case it was free, and a 'social care' bath – provided by a home help, in which case you might need to pay towards it. A distinction utterly irrelevant of course to the person who just needs help to have a bath. Despite many efforts to improve the way the NHS and social care work together, there remain too many examples of people falling between the cracks of the NHS and social care, of having to tell their stories over and over again to different professionals and struggling to understand why they have to pay for some kinds of help themselves while other services are free.

For people with intensive clinical needs, such as a high level of nursing care, it is even worse. They face a further hurdle of being assessed as to whether those needs are so great as to qualify for 'continuing healthcare' (discussed later). If they are, the NHS will meet the full costs, including the full cost of social care. The financial consequences for the individual can be huge, and the process utterly dispiriting. Continuing healthcare is arguably the worst example of a disjointed health and care system. It is one of the darkest places in the British welfare state.

There have also been some big changes in who provides care. From the 1980s onwards, more and more services, particularly care homes and home care services, were outsourced to voluntary and private bodies. In many cases, councils themselves transferred their own services to newly created independent organisations because it was cheaper and because they could borrow money to make essential building improvements, to meet regulatory standards, in a way that councils could not. This has been a mixed blessing. It replaced councils' accountability to the local electorate for its services with control exercised through a commercial contract. The new 'market' in care made possible the entry of major private equity companies. Many have complex and opaque funding structures and high levels of debt and were necessarily driven by shareholders seeking high profits. The collapse of the Southern Cross nursing home chain in 2011 was an early warning sign. Gone are the days when councils routinely constructed purpose-built care homes and wore these programmes as a badge of civic pride, a measure of how well they looked after their senior citizens. The wholesale outsourcing of care over the last 40 years has taken place by stealth and has attracted little debate and few headlines (Hudson, 2021). In comparison, the relatively modest use of private hospitals to provide NHS care has provoked uproar.

The risks of outsourcing were made worse by cash-strapped councils bearing down on the fees they pay to providers and fuelling financial instability. Providers complain that councils are not paying them enough to meet the full cost of care which meets the standards set down by their regulator, the Care Quality Commission (setting aside that fact that establishing the true cost of care is far from straightforward and can vary, for legitimate reasons, from place to place). Councils retort that they pay what they can afford and do so with some justification. Despite recent cash boosts, councils' spending on social care in 2020 barely exceeded what they spent in 2010 because of severe cuts in financial support from the government earlier in the decade. (Bottery and Ward, 2021). Some care homes plug the gap by levying higher charges on those residents who pay for their own care – 41 per cent more according to one estimate – but this is not an option for those in poorer areas with few 'self-funders' (Competition and Markets Authority, 2017). COVID-19 has made things worse because of higher costs – for infection control, personal protective equipment and staffing cover – and falling income. It is no wonder that 60 per cent of local social care chiefs report that, in just six months, providers in their area have closed, ceased trading or handed back contracts (ADASS, 2020). The market in social care has never been more fragile and precarious. The government has little awareness of how well the market is working or the effectiveness of services that are commissioned by councils, although, in response to COVID-19, work is underway to obtain better data and implement a new assurance framework to assess council performance (NAO, 2021).

In 2020, the independent ombudsman described a 'staggering' 72 per cent rise in the number of complaints about social care in which it found fault, leading it to conclude that adult social care is 'progressively failing to deliver for those who need it most': 'Increasingly it is a system where exceptional and sometimes unorthodox measures are being deployed simply to balance the books – a reality we see frequently pleaded in their defence by the councils and care providers we investigate' (Local Government and Social Care Ombudsman, 2021).

Who cares?

If any further evidence is needed of just how far our social care arrangements have fallen behind, look no further than the people who work in social care. In the eyes of people who use social care, they *are* the service, and the quality of the relationship with the care worker is what defines their experience of social care.

A few years ago, in my mother-in-law's home town in Sweden, there was an outcry about the use of migrant workers in care services. The outcry was less about them being migrants, but that they might not be paid and trained to Swedish standards. The comparison with England, with its dismal picture of low pay and poor investment in training, could not be starker. In the year before COVID-19 struck, there were 112,000 care job vacancies at any one time; 440,000 people were leaving their job each year; the turnover rate was over 30 per cent; and one third of these were leaving the sector completely. A quarter of staff were employed on zero-hours contracts. The average pay was £8.10 per hour. In some parts of the country, as many as 13 per cent of adult social care jobs were filled by EU nationals, jeopardised by the uncertain impact of Brexit (Skills for Care, 2019). The requirement from November 2021 that all staff working in care services must have full vaccination against COVID19 – 'no jab, no job' – could, by the government's own estimates, see the loss of anything between 17,000 and 70,000 workers from the sector (DHSC, 2021). With the policy set to be extended to the NHS, concerns about the impact on staffing led to a government U-turn in February 2021. But this came too late to prevent a haemorrhaging of staff from social care services. In future years, even more staff will be needed – another 480,000 by 2035 if present trends continue (Skills for Care, 2021).

Yet there is no national plan or strategy as to how we will tackle this malaise or where those half a million new workers will come from. In its annual assessment of the state of care, the Care Quality Commission warned that the workforce shortages were 'serious and deteriorating' (Care Quality Commission, 2021). Of all aspects of the crisis in social care, this is the most worrying and most immediate. It goes deeper than the statistics, which themselves do not capture just how little care work is valued and recognised. In her book *Labour of Love*, Madeleine Bunting interviewed employees in a variety of 'care' settings, from care homes to GP surgeries and even in the back of an ambulance. She describes how the essential qualities of care are about the relationships between people, the bonds of interdependency that unite us, and the essential values of kindness and altruism.

Qualities that struggle for air in a climate of cost reduction, understaffing and low pay (Bunting, 2020).

The human costs

The crisis in social care is framed not just by the metrics of spreadsheets and charts, but by its impact on the lives of everyone involved in providing and receiving care. It is remarkable that, despite all these problems and pressures, people who use social care generally appear to be very satisfied with the care they receive. Stories abound about the good that social care does, of lives changed, people protected. But there are some important caveats. There are still too many examples of poor-quality care and people who have been let down badly by the system that was supposed to be looking after them. This is not always due to lack of money. We know little about the experience of people who pay for their own care but what we do know is not encouraging, with many struggling to find their way around a complex system (Henwood et al, 2020). It seems absurd that, instead of designing something easy for people to use, we have ended up with a system so complicated and bewildering that some places have created a new type of worker called a 'care navigator' to help people to use it. Getting into the system in the first place is not straightforward. Although the old Victorian institutions that housed elderly, disabled and destitute people, with forbidding walls designed to keep people in, have long gone, modern social care has constructed new, virtual walls that, if anything, are designed to keep people out, spawning a vocabulary of 'gatekeeping' (requiring gatekeepers), eligibility, thresholds and pathways, signposting and demand management. Alex Fox likens it to 'an exclusive nightclub with huge bouncers and an unfathomable door policy, but once inside it is disappointing and hard to find your way out of' (Fox, 2018).

Social care is described as a 'system', yet the reality for too many people is a random collection of uncoordinated cogs and wheels that grind together. It is a wonder that so many people receive good care and that there are, as Sara Ryan puts it, 'pockets of brilliance amongst the mediocrity' (Ryan, 2020).

These successes are achieved despite 'the system' not because of it, arising from the commitment, kindness and basic human decency of individual members of staff.

Beyond the fractures of funding and services, there is a fundamental challenge arising from the fact that different people want different things from social care, reflecting the enormous diversity of individual circumstances discussed earlier. Anna Severwright, a former doctor in her 30s, now co-convenor of the #SocialCareFuture movement who has used social care for many years, describes her experiences:

> I get 31 hours a week of social care, of which 20 are for things like personal care and food preparation. They are the things that are keeping me fed, clean and watered. There are just under 12 hours of social inclusion, which, effectively, is the bit for me to be able to go out. I live by myself, so I need support to get about. As someone in my 30s, that is not a lot of time. If, in the evening, I think. 'Oh, I'd like to go and meet up with so-and-so', that spontaneity is completely not there. I have to plan well ahead, even down to what time I go food shopping. I need to know that I have a PA (Personal Assistant) who can come with me. It has a big impact on my sense of self. I spend an awful lot of time at home by myself, quite lonely and quite fed up. (Health and Social Care Committee, 2020a)

Anna's words sum up the difference between wanting a life and receiving a service. They exemplify how the aspirations and expectations of today's users of social care are different from and higher than their predecessors (though we should not assume that new cohorts of older people with care needs will share the tendency of many of their predecessors to be grateful for whatever they are offered). It's not enough to be kept 'fed, clean and watered.' Rightly, they want to be active participants in deciding and shaping their own care and support, not passive recipients of traditional services. For those who provide care, the shrinkage of support to basic 'life and limb' care is dispiriting, as Marie, a care home manager, explains:

> For older people, especially, our offer can be very basic and limited. It isn't about quality of life. It's about making sure somebody is clean and making sure they are fed. That takes the joy out of care work. It's hard for people to do that job. It is not a valued job. (Butler, 2021)

There is also a growing sense that, as budgets have tightened, social care has become distracted by processes that are more about the needs of organisations than the people they serve. Kate Sibthorp's daughter has learning disabilities and autism and is supported by a team of personal assistants. She obtained funding so one of them could go to college to get a Certificate in Care:

> She decided to abandon it after just two weeks. She was being told that she had to record in writing, every day, exactly what they'd done – how many drinks, how many visits to the loo etc. She told the course tutor that I didn't want to know these things. I wanted to know if my daughter had had a good day – was she happy, had people been friendly, would she enjoy going back to wherever they'd been or seeing a film again. The tutor said that the PA should still write everything down to 'cover herself' in case of a problem situation. It was all process, not relationships or happiness. The only way anyone could measure what matters for my daughter would be to count smiles and laughter. The relationship between me, my daughter and her PAs is built on trust. Sometimes the PA might do something I wouldn't have done, but if it's coming from the right place, the heart, that's fine. And anyway, who's to say the PA's 'wrong' and I'm 'right'? I'm happy for them to try things and see whether my daughter likes them or not. (Sibthorp, 2020)

For many people, the experience of being assessed for social care is decidedly mixed. Jessica Thom has care and support needs arising from Tourette's syndrome that was diagnosed in her 20s.

She describes her approach to social services for an assessment in 2011 as 'life changing' and 'one of the best decisions' she has ever made. Her memories of that first assessment were positive, dubbing the assessor 'London's best social worker' (reflecting the enduring importance and power of relationships in social care):

> It was thorough, clear and left me feeling cared about – this was 2011, before the impact of austerity had really begun to bite. I've had many social care reviews since then, some more difficult than others. The stakes are always incredibly high. With the right support I can live a happy, full, independent life and feel safe most of the time. Without it, everything that makes me 'me' is on the line. (Thom, 2021)

More recently, she observed that:

> Despite everyone's best efforts, the assessment process can feel pretty brutal. It's a very in-depth process with requirements assessed across twelve different areas of care. Weirdly it's not straightforwardly about assessing whether I need support, or what this support should be. Both the NHS assessor and my social worker agree that I need support and would be at serious risk without it. What this is ultimately about is who should pay for it – social services or health? It's simultaneously about me and my support requirements, and not about me at all. It puts me in the weird position of explaining my requirements in detail, and then standing back as the health worker and social worker debate where I come on a scale from low to severe. It's the closest you can get to knowing what it feels like to be an antique being haggled over on *Bargain Hunt*.

These perspectives raise big questions, rarely asked in many of the formal discussions and debates, about what is the purpose of social care in our fast-changing 21st-century society? What is it for? Who should do it and how? How do we pay for it? There is no single or 'right' set of answers to these questions, instead our personal views will be shaped by our circumstances, needs and values. In turn, these are underpinned by an essentially political and values-driven view of what is a good society. While everyone agrees that something should be done about social care, there is no consensus about *what* should be done. Perhaps it is easier to plunge into the technocratic minutiae of funding options than grapple with these fundamental issues about purpose and values.

To summarise, the crisis in social care arises from multiple problems to do with 'hard' issues like how it is funded, staffed and organised, but underpinned by 'soft' issues such as changing needs and expectations and a sense that we have lost touch with the essence of what caring for each other is all about. There is a widespread perception that the altruistic basis of social care as a public service has been compromised by organisational needs to balance budgets and ration care. Some, but not all, of these problems have been recognised by governments of all political persuasions. In England since 1997, these issues have received the variable attention of five prime ministers, ten secretaries of state for health and fifteen ministers for care services. Much blood, sweat and tears has been expended by policy-makers in producing around 13 White Papers, Green Papers and formal consultations. There have been at least five independent reviews of funding. Bookshelves groan with one report after another describing different aspects of the problem and analysing possible solutions. Yet for too many people too little has changed. For an example of an issue where successive governments have left things undone that sorely needed to be done, look no further. In September 2021, the government announced its long-awaited plan for social care entitled 'Build Back Better: Our plan for health and social care', accompanied two months later by a long-awaited White Paper, 'People at the Heart of Care', setting out wider plans for reform (HM Government, 2021; DHSC, 2021c). Both documents will be considered later in more detail.

Why I wrote this book

I've spent a decade at the King's Fund analysing the problem of funding and options to deal with it. I have advised commissions and enquiries, including the Barker Commission and the House of Lords Economic Affairs Committee. I spent many years as a local authority director and assistant director of social services trying to make the pieces of the jigsaw fit together, and trying hard not to forget what attracted me to a career in social work some two decades earlier. In writing this book, I have drawn on hundreds and thousands of conversations over the years with people who work in social care and in the NHS – people who provide it and those who commission it; people who take on caring roles, for love, money and often both; the countless organisations, large and small, national and local, who exist to campaign and work for better social care. For many years during my time at the Department of Health, the conversations involved civil servants, ministers and their advisors. And my local government career left me in no doubt about the frustrations of elected councillors charged with local responsibility for social care but feeling that they have little control or influence over the national levers of finance and policy.

The trigger that finally compelled me to write this book was my personal experience in sorting out care for my late father. This brought me into close personal contact with the best and worst of our social care system. The best was that the final years of my father's life were good ones, thanks to superb person-centred residential care that gave him his life back after months of pain and misery in that rose-tinted place called the community. The worst was the battle with the cash-strapped local authority when his money began to run out, insisting that wrenching him away from the place he called his home, in the community where he had lived for over 25 years, to a cheaper home the other side of the county, would not damage his wellbeing. So much for the Care Act principle of that name.

It left me feeling a stranger to the system in which I had worked for over 40 years. None of my extensive experience and knowledge was enough to prepare me for the bruising, adversarial series of encounters that were to come with the officialdom that is supposed to serve the public not fight with it. Four years on, I am deeply troubled, as a former social worker and director of social services, to write these words. I was left thinking that if it were like this for me, a so-called expert and seasoned social care professional, what on earth must it be like for those with none of my advantages? We use the expression 'expert by experience' to denote those whose expertise comes from substantial lived experience of social care. For me, it felt like I had become an 'expert by inexperience'. Conversations with friends and colleagues from a similar background sadly confirmed that my experience was not a one-off. The crisis in social care is not a single calamitous national event but the invisible accretion of many thousands of individual crises experienced in homes, hospitals and other places throughout the land. How, and why, has it come to this? Time inexorably moves us all closer to the point when we, or someone close to us, may need social care for ourselves. The professional becomes the personal and the personal is the political.

It caused me to reflect on the conundrum that our social care system has in some ways remained strangely insulated from the forces of human progress that have transformed so many aspects of our lives for the better. In recent times, for example, we have witnessed the brilliance of human ingenuity in rapidly producing vaccines against COVID-19 and genomic mapping techniques that can very quickly identify mutant strains of the virus so we can tackle it quickly. We can send a spacecraft 293 million miles to the surface of Mars. The smart phones many of us carry out in our pockets have 100,000 times more computer power than *Apollo 11* that landed men on the moon nearly 50 years ago. Meanwhile, the basic need to give and receive care has been a feature of the human condition since the dawn of time. The goal of a humane, effective and sustainable care system – something that is set to touch the lives of millions of us – continues to defy resolution and in some respects we have gone backwards. Why that is so, and more importantly what can be done about it, is the central theme of this book.

How this book is structured

Having outlined the main problems of the social care system in England, the underlying issues and challenges behind the crisis in social care are examined. Although much of this discussion is relevant to all parts of the UK, responsibility for social care policy sits with the devolved administrations of Northern Ireland, Scotland and Wales. They are pursuing an increasingly different approach to reform (see, for example, Oung et al, 2020) and for that reason the focus of this book is on England.

Chapter 2 describes how we got here – a brief history of social care since 1948; the dramatic changes in the nature and volume of needs that need to be met; the impact of changes in health care; the implications of the growth in property ownership and personal wealth; and the key policy and organisational developments, including funding changes, the withdrawal of the NHS from long-term care and the outsourcing of services.

Chapter 3 aims to explain the social care system we have today – what we mean by social care, who gets it, how it is supposed to work and the financial resources – public and private – involved. The economic significance of the sector is highlighted and the importance of other separate streams of public money aimed at care needs – what is described as 'the social care pound'.

Chapter 4 examines the efforts of successive governments since the 1990s to reform social care. With so little to show for the procession of reviews, commissions, White Papers and Green Papers over the years, what are the lessons we should learn and what are the implications for the politics and process of reform? Chapter 5 looks at the experience of other advanced countries that have successfully reformed social care, with lessons that can be learned and potentially applied to England.

Chapter 6 focuses on the workforce aspects of the social care crisis and develops further the introduction's analysis. It examines the nuanced nature of caring and the importance of relationships and reciprocity in good social care. It sketches out some short-term and longer-range ideas as part of a 'people plan' for adult social care that would secure a skilled, valued and well-paid workforce for the future.

The book then looks to the future and argues that a comprehensive range of reforms to social care funding, delivery and entitlements is needed, on a scale akin to the creation of the NHS in 1948. Instead of trying to 'build back better' on the shaky foundations of the current arrangements, the aim should be to design a new social care system that is fit for the 21st century.

Chapter 7 argues that a different road to reform is needed to secure political traction and public support for change. This would involve replacing traditional, top-down policy-making with a new approach, using the principles of co-production, deliberative democracy, consensus-building and drawing on new thinking about long-term policy-making.

The final chapter sets out three building blocks of a new system. These are rooted in the new reality that all advanced countries depend on good social care as part of their economic and social infrastructure, in the same way that they depend on investments in education, skills and health care. The three building blocks are:

1. a new social 'contract for care' that sets out the mutual roles and responsibilities of individuals, families, communities and the state (national and local), based on the simple truth that most of us will give and receive support at some point on our lives;
2. a different model of design and delivery that gives people new rights and resources to shape the care and support arrangements that work for all of us; offers peace of mind to everyone who needs care now, or will do so in the future; and secures a new deal for people who provide care and support, both paid and unpaid;
3. a new funding settlement that positions social care as a major public service in its own right, on a par with other universal services such as education and health care.

One thing that has changed for the better in recent years is the increasing recognition of listening to and engaging with people who have experience of social care. Most chapters in this book include examples from such experience, including my own. These illustrate the best and worst of the 'system' and also offer some powerful pointers to what better social care should look like.

2

A brief history: how we got here

The social service movement of modern times is not confined to any one class, nor is it the preserve of a particular section of dull and respectable people. It has arisen out of a deep discontent with society as at present constituted, and among its prophets have been the greatest spirits of our time. It is not a movement concerned alone with the material, with housing and drains, clinics and feeding centres, gas and water, but is the expression of the desire for social justice, for freedom and beauty, and for the better apportionment of all the things that make up a good life.

Clement Attlee, *The Social Worker* (1920)

In need of care and attention – the 1940s

The need to care for each other has been a universal human need since the start of recorded time. It has found expression down the ages in the work of monasteries, medieval almshouses and the earliest hospitals that were essentially places of refuge, care and support. The Elizabethan and Victorian Poor Laws marked the beginnings of state intervention in response to the plight of the poor, the destitute and those unable to care for themselves. The motives for these measures were often more punitive than philanthropic, but they have left their mark, as we shall see.

To understand how we have ended up with our current system, the starting point for the modern history of social care should be the foundations of the post-war welfare state, when the social security element of the Poor Law was shifted to central government (social security as it was to be called later), and the 'welfare' element was given to new welfare departments within local authorities. This was a decisive moment that was to influence deeply the relationship between social care and its very big and dominant sibling, the NHS. Looking back to the origins of the modern welfare state also helps us to appreciate how much, and in many ways how little, has changed since then.

In the early months of 1948, a leaflet by the Ministry of Health plopped through the letterbox of every household in the land, proclaiming the launch of the new National Health Service on 5 July:

> It will provide you with all medical, dental and nursing care. Everyone – rich or poor, man, woman or child-can use it or any part of it. There are no charges, except for a few special items. There are no insurance qualifications. But it is not a 'charity'. You are all paying for it, mainly as taxpayers, and it will relieve your money worries in time of illness.

The benefits of the new service, to individuals and to society, were expressed more lyrically by its founding father, Nye Bevan: 'Society becomes more wholesome, more serene, spiritually healthier, if it knows that its citizens haver at the back of their consciousness the knowledge that not only themselves, but all their fellows, have access, when ill, to the best that medical skill can offer' (Foot, 2009).

Thus began the nation's love affair with the NHS, universally available, free at the point of use and not based on ability to pay – principles and a relationship that has endured in good times and bad.

But if the NHS was a bright new dawn for health care, it was a different story for people with non-medical care and support needs – what today we call social care. In the same year as the NHS began to great fanfare, its sister legislation, the National Assistance Act quietly slid onto the statute book and was to serve as the legal cornerstone of social care for the next 66 years. Its opening words, 'An Act to eliminate the Poor Law ...', could not offer more of a contrast with that upbeat promise in the Ministry of Health leaflet. The 1948 act placed a duty on local authorities to 'provide residential accommodation for persons who by reason of age, infirmity or other circumstances are in need of care and attention which is not otherwise available to them.' It talked about 'welfare arrangements for blind, deaf, dumb and crippled persons', which was to underpin the core definition of disability for the purposes of community care law for the next 66 years (Law Commission, 2011). These were very limited duties, and it was not until the 1970 Chronically Sick and Disabled Persons Act that councils were given the power to offer a wider range of support.

These new duties in 1948 were the responsibility of new local authority welfare departments (there were separate departments for mental health and for children) whose staff were mostly unqualified. Many had worked under the old Poor Law. This organisational architecture of separate departments was to remain largely unchanged until 1970. It helps to explain why the influence of the Victorian Poor Law, based on notions of 'deserving' and 'undeserving poor' and 'less eligibility' have had such a pervasive influence on social care for such a long time. As a young social worker in the late 1970s, I can recall reassuring a very anxious lady in her 80s that moving into a modern local authority care home was not the same as entering the workhouse. To help allay her fears and persuade her to pay an introductory visit, I used the unusual social work technique of photography to show her pictures of the brand-new purpose-built home.

The 1948 act also placed a legal duty on councils to recover payments from a person provided with residential accommodation and to assess their ability to pay if they were unable to pay the full cost. This cemented into place the means-testing regime that remains to this day.

It is perhaps ironic that the prime minister who oversaw the foundation of the welfare state, Clem Attlee, was originally a social worker with a keen understanding of the relationship between social work, wider social conditions and social justice (Attlee, 1920). Yet the extent to which the NHS was established on a completely different basis from what in 1948 was called 'national assistance' has reverberated down the years with three enduring consequences that have deepened the fractures between the NHS and social care, despite much rhetoric about integrating health and social care.

The first is that, despite the introduction of some charges, most NHS care remains free at the point of use, and it aims, albeit with mixed success, to cater for a wide range of needs, from ingrowing toenails to complex neurosurgery. Attempts to introduce new charges or increase existing ones have been fiercely resisted. Social care by contrast is heavily means tested and has been ever since 1948. Even the big overhaul of social care law that that produced the Care Act in 2014 left means testing in place. Part 2 of the act would it have made it more generous, but implementation of this was postponed in 2015 and later abandoned altogether. Means testing is one of the deepest fault lines between the NHS and social care.

From the outset, social care was never intended to be a universal service meeting a wide range of needs like the NHS. It offered only a safety net, with councils having very limited powers and duties to provide particular services. In recent years, care has been increasingly restricted to those with the very highest needs as a result of council budget pressures. Imagine being told by your GP that your minor but painful ailment is not severe enough to be eligible for NHS treatment and to come back when it got worse. Or that you have to bear a large portion of the cost of your surgery because your savings exceed the threshold for public funding. These are everyday scenarios for people with care and support needs. That is not to say that rationing in the NHS does not exist, or that some of us have to pay for some things such as prescriptions or dental charges, but the scale of eligibility for its services is far greater than social care and almost all clinical care is free at the point of use. Any suggestion that access to free NHS care should be limited only to those with the highest needs and the lowest means would be greeted with outrage. (In 1958, the prospect of introducing hotel and other charges promoted the resignation of three Conservative ministers.) Whereas most people would regard rich people getting free emergency care on the NHS as an expression of social solidarity, proposals for free, or more generous, social care are opposed on the grounds that poorer taxpayers should not be funding the care of better-off people who can afford to pay for it themselves. The application of a different political or moral calculus to entitlements to social care compared with health care has been a great obstacle to placing the former on the same basis as the latter.

A second consequence follows on from the sheer universality of the NHS. Everyone uses it, irrespective of wealth or class, and at some point in our lives, especially at the beginning and the end, all of us will. Over eight decades, its presence and familiarity has been deeply embedded in our national culture and identity, lauded in the opening ceremony of the London Olympics in 2012 and manifested more recently in the clap for carers every Thursday night during the early months of COVID-19. Observers from other countries were nonplussed by exhortations to 'Protect the NHS' when it was thought the NHS was there to protect the people (Castle, 2020). No wonder former chancellor Nigel Lawson described the NHS as the closest thing the English have to a national religion, though that might have come as a surprise to the Church of England.

We know what the NHS is, where it is, and how it gets paid for. The blue and white NHS lozenge is a powerful brand, on the door and on the documents of every hospital, clinic and GP surgery in the country. The popularity and familiarity of the NHS has made it politically sacrosanct. Even those on the right of the political spectrum who favour markets and private insurance have largely given up any serious prospect of prising the British public away from its deep affection for the NHS, despite occasional noises-off.

It is not surprising that the nation's love affair for the NHS has caused many to see the solution to social care as making it more like the NHS, by creating a National Care Service, as proposed by the Labour government in 2010 or more recently by an independent review in Scotland, or even integrating it with the NHS altogether. There has even been an attempt to ape the famous NHS logo with an equivalent 'CARE' badge described by a previous Secretary of State as "a badge of honour in a very real sense, allowing social care staff proudly and publicly to identify themselves, just like NHS staff do with that famous blue and white logo" (DHSC, 2020). But so far these have been largely cosmetic and emotional aspirations, with little appetite for giving social care parity of funding and entitlements.

A third consequence of the 1948 settlement was to bequeath yet another set of dividing lines between the two services in how they were run, to whom they were accountable and how they were funded. For the NHS, the key word in this respect is 'National'. The Secretary of State is accountable to Parliament for the NHS; there is a single financial settlement coming from general taxation. Local NHS bodies are accountable upwards through regional tiers to a national overseeing body. Currently this is NHS England, though the titles and tiers of organisations have changed many times over the years. In contrast, welfare services in 1948, and therefore social care today, are the responsibility of local authorities. The key word is 'local'. Councillors are elected by and accountable to local people and each council makes local decisions about spending and services. There is no national financial settlement for social care. Instead, it relies on a mix of local and national taxes and grants – a complex combination that has changed over the years (discussed in more detail in the next chapter). These fundamental differences in governance, funding and accountability have bedevilled attempts to get the NHS and social care to work together more closely. It does not help that local government in England has been weakened by recent decades of centralisation in which more powers and decisions have been moved to central government (see, for example, Bogdanor, 1999).

In short, the way social care works today and many of its challenges reflect the different tramlines laid down in 1948 and its origins in the Victorian Poor Law that predated the welfare state.

In sickness and in health

Life was not only very different in 1948 but much shorter. Life expectancy at birth was just above the state pension retirement age of 65. There were just over 750,000 people aged over 80 – just a quarter of the number today. There was no great expectation that many people would live long enough to need much care. The country had just come through a world war in which the Home Office had calculated 20 million feet of timber would be needed every month for coffins (Harrisson, 1976). At least half a million lives had been lost. The prospect of peace and survival, and then reconstruction, was more than enough. Increased life expectancy was not exactly uppermost in everyone's minds. Yet today it is 79 years for men and 82.9 for women. Much of this is due to dramatic improvements in infant mortality. In 1940, there were around 61 infant deaths per 1,000 live births, but, by 2006, the figure had dropped to just 5 per 1,000. In 2019, it was 3.7 (ONS, 2021e). Although there are signs that the steady increase in life expectancy throughout this and the last century has stalled, or fallen back slightly because of COVID-19, the older population is increasing faster than other age groups. Projections are that, by 2050, one in four people in the UK will be aged 65 and over. Over the next 20 years, the number of people aged 85 and over – the group with the greatest needs for social care – is set to double (ONS, 2019).

It easy to overlook what a success story this has been. Who has not heard the story that the Queen now has to employ a team of seven people to send telegrams (telegrams?) to people on their 100th birthday? It is hard to keep up with the steady flow of books and articles about our ageing population. Camilla Cavendish's *Extra Time* and Anna Dixon's *The Age of Ageing Better* are notable additions to the genre, both full of ideas about the opportunities our longer lives bring, providing we rise to the policy challenges (Cavendish, 2019, Dixon, 2020). But instead of recognising and celebrating longevity, much of the media coverage and policy debate exhibits a lazy pessimism that depicts ageing in terms of decline, dependency, a financial burden on younger people of working age (as though no one over 65 works any more) and a tsunami of need that will overwhelm the public finances. Many of the policy documents that litter the history of social care refer to the 'dependency ratio' – the number of older people as a percentage of those of working age – with the insinuation that increasing numbers of older people are placing a strain on the taxes and finances of the younger population. It is nowhere near as simple as that. The dependency ratio makes no allowance for the many ways in which older people continue to contribute to society through employment, volunteering and child care, but the language of dependency illustrates the tendency to see ageing as a problem rather than an opportunity.

The big improvement in life expectancy since 1948 is closely linked to portentous changes in the pattern of illness – the 'burden of disease' in the technical argot of epidemiologists – since 1948. Dementia has displaced infectious diseases as a leading cause of deaths. Better treatment means that more people are surviving diseases like cancer, stroke and heart disease and living longer. The most striking change in the nation's health in the last century is the steady rise in chronic illness. Around 18 million adults have long-term health conditions, ranging from depression to diabetes. Over half of older people have at least two such conditions – the challenge of multimorbidity, which rises more steeply the older we get. The numbers of older people with at least four long-term health conditions are set to double between 2015 and 2035 (Kingston et al, 2018). There is a strong overlap between physical health and mental health needs, and many people with long-term health problems will have care and support needs as well. If Nye Bevan were alive today, he would be astonished that long-term health conditions account for £7 of every £10 spent on health and care (Department of Health, 2012). His belief that the demand for health care would fall as the backlog of medical need was cleared by the new NHS was quickly disabused.

The combined effect of these changes is a dramatic and continuing increase in the numbers of us that will need care and support at all ages. It is not just about older people. Advances in medical care mean that children born with complex health issues have much better chances of survival, and many children with disabilities live well into adulthood, although, shockingly, the life expectancy of people with a learning disability is at least 14 years lower than the general population (NHS Digital, 2020). Forty per cent of people aged 50 to 59 have at least one long-term health condition, as do a quarter of 40–49-year-olds. There has been a steady growth in the proportion of younger adults reporting a disability, rising from 14 per cent in 2007–08 to 18 per cent in 2017–18. When combined with population growth, the number of younger adults with a self-reported disability has risen by around 35 per cent, compared with around 16 per cent in the older age group.

These trends help to explain why the need for social care has increased faster among 18–64-year-olds in recent years. This is set to continue. Over the next 20 years, 29 per cent more 18–64-year-olds will have a care and support need. For people with learning disabilities, the increase is a staggering 72 per cent (Wittenberg et al 2018). Younger adults with care needs generally receive more intensive support. Almost half of younger adults have continuous support, compared with a third of older people, and their needs are often more expensive to meet (Idriss et al, 2020).

Apart from the obvious financial implications, these trends suggest four conclusions about the kind of social care we need in the future. The first is that people need a mixture of help from a range of different services. Yet our health and care system still operates through old silos that, despite multiple reorganisations, have survived largely intact since the 1940s – among them hospital care, general practice, community health and social care services, and mental health services. The rhetoric of integrated care is still not a reality for many. The poor coordination of services is a persistent complaint by many who use health and social care. It was summed up by one the experts by experience who advised the Barker Commission:

> I know how the system is supposed to work, but I was powerless to influence Mam's care at a distance. Nothing was joined-up, with each part of the system only interested in their part of the problem. Primary, secondary and social care all worked separately, with the former two needing as much attention on integration as latter. (Commission on the Future of Health and Social Care in England, 2014)

There have been many attempts over the last 40 years to bring services closer together. Integrated care systems are the latest answer to the question of how we ensure people get joined-up care (Charles, 2021). This is important because people with social care needs, especially those that live in care homes, are much more likely to have clinical needs. The acuity of needs in all settings is much higher than was the case 30 years ago, with care workers routinely expected to carry out tasks that years ago would have been done by nurses.

The second conclusion to be drawn from these trends is that a modern social care system should address the needs and aspirations of people of all ages and not just older people. Yet so much of the policy and media debate in recent years assumes that social care is only about the latter.

The third conclusion is that the demands made of social care, and the health service too, can be greatly reduced if economic and social conditions make it easier for people live healthy and fulfilled lives, and if people are supported to live well with their illness and disability. Ensuring that we spend more of our longer lives in good health and independence – healthy life expectancy – is a vital policy objective. This relatively new concept of population health has profound implications for the kind of social care system we need (King's Fund, 2019), and will be considered in more detail in Chapter 8.

The final conclusion is that, irrespective of our age, there are many more of us. The UK's population has burgeoned from 49 million in 1948 to 67 million in 2019. By 2031, it will pass 69 million, reaching 71 million by 2045 (ONS, 2022). Much of the growth since the 1990s has been due to migration, a phenomenon that has generally been good news for social care.

Going private

Our ageing population, and its implications, gets plenty of media coverage, in the form of advertising pitched at wealthy baby boomers or doom-laden prophecies about the unaffordability of pensions and health care. Some momentous changes, however, have happened quietly and with little discussion or public awareness. Back in 1948, people needing long-term care would most likely get it in an NHS hospital. The NHS was then a major provider of long-term care for older people and those with learning disabilities and mental illness, through a network of long-stay institutions, many of which were former workhouse buildings. In addition, many of the municipal and local hospitals the NHS inherited in 1948 had geriatric wards. The sheer scale of this provision meant that many people were able to receive free long-term care under the NHS, avoiding the means-testing clutches of local authorities. I can remember in the 1970s accompanying my mother to visit a close family friend, Dora, who lived for over 15 years in the geriatric ward of a local Victorian hospital, a former workhouse, after a catastrophic cerebral haemorrhage in her early 50s. The quality of her physical care seemed good, but, without visitors, she spent most of her time in a void of silence and isolation. As late as 1960, 34,000 older people were still resident in former workhouse buildings (Townsend, 1964).

Since then, the NHS has dramatically reduced the number of general and acute hospital beds – from just under 400,000 in the 1970s to around 141,000 today. The closure of long-stay institutions for people with mental health and learning disabilities accounts for some, but not all, of this. There have been big reductions in the numbers of long-term beds for older people, accounting for most of the 44 per cent fall in general and acute hospital beds since 1987–88 – the geriatric back-wards that were home for people like Dora. In 1987, there were over 53,000 beds for older people. By 2009, it had dropped to just under 21,000 (Ewbank et al, 2021). The NHS has largely withdrawn from providing long-term care. Today, Dora would almost certainly have been transferred from the acute hospital to an independently run nursing home, hopefully with an intervening period of rehabilitation or intermediate care. An assessment would determine whether her health care needs were sufficiently significant and ongoing to qualify for 'continuing healthcare', in which case the NHS would pay for all her care needs – medical and social. Otherwise, depending on her financial circumstances, she or the council would have to pick up the bill. Around 55,000 people receive continuing healthcare funded by the NHS (compared with around 840,000 people whose care is funded by their local council), a number that has reduced significantly since 2017 despite population growth (NHS England, 2021).

The point here is that responsibility for long-term care over several decades has shifted almost by stealth from the free-at-the-point-of-use NHS to the means-tested social care system. The bill for care that previously would have been met by the NHS is now picked up either by councils or individuals and sometimes both. There has been little discussion or debate about whether this shift was right or fair.

There have been other ways in which the boundary between the NHS and social care has shifted over the years. One reason the NHS has been able to reduce bed numbers is that medical advances have reduced the amount of time we need to spend in hospital. In 1998–99, the average length of stay in English hospitals was just over 8 days. By 2018–19, that had nearly halved to 4.5 days. There has also been a dramatic increase in the number of procedures that no longer require a hospital stay but can be performed as day cases, for example in ear, nose, throat and cataract surgery (Ewbank et al, 2021).

One effect of reducing the length of hospital stays is that the recuperative or convalescent element of a person's recovery, where needed, no longer happens in hospital but at home, with responsibility for care shifting to the family, or, for those with no family, to social care services.

Many of these changes have been beneficial in so many ways. NHS capacity has been properly reserved for increases in acute and emergency demand. And no one mourns the passing of long-stay institutions and geriatric back-wards. In his famous 'water towers' speech in 1961, a junior health minister by the name of Enoch Powell conveyed the impact of the old asylums with a lyricism rarely found in ministerial speeches, hinting at the difficulties still experienced today in shifting care away from buildings:

> There they stand, isolated, majestic, imperious, brooded over by the gigantic water-tower and chimney combined, rising unmistakable and daunting out of the countryside – the asylums which our forefathers built with such immense solidity – to express the notions of their day. Do not for a moment underestimate their powers of resistance to our assault. (Enoch Powell, cited in Rivet G, 2019)

There was no golden age of long-term care under the NHS, as a succession of scandals involving poor conditions and abuse, from the 1970s to the present day, have demonstrated only too well. Indeed, modern, well-designed and well-led care homes offer a quality of care that is so much better, and for most people the right combination of housing and care support is better still. Spending less time in hospital is generally a good thing, to avoid infection, deconditioning and depression. These changes have enabled the NHS to treat more patients, quicker and with fewer beds.

But the impact of these changes on social care, except for the closure of the institutions, was never anticipated, quantified or planned for. In fact, it has been 20 years since the NHS last took a proper look at how many beds it needs, what they are used for, and the implications for other services like GPs, district nurses and social care. It illustrates a concept that health economists call the 'substitution' effect – in this context, when one kind of care resource is reduced or unavailable, the need will fall somewhere else, typically family carers, social care, GP and district nursing services (Fernandez and Forder, 2011).

Because the UK has fewer acute beds relative to its population than many comparable health systems, the pressure on beds has become intense. Occupancy levels before COVID-19 regularly exceeded 95 per cent and the winter beds crisis has become a problem all year round. It produces one of the most controversial flashpoints in how the NHS works with social care, the problem of 'delayed transfers of care'[1] – people who are medically fit to be discharged, but are stuck in hospital waiting for follow-up care. This will be explored further in the next chapter.

The withdrawal of the NHS from long-term care and other changes are examples of the powerful and often unintentional impact the NHS has had in shaping the contours of our social care system. There was another change over 40 years ago that was decisive in shaping what today we call the social care 'market'.

In the 1970s, voluntary-run hostels and care homes, under the cosh of severe public expenditure cuts, began to persuade local social security offices to make 'board and lodging payments' for their residents. This was subsequently codified in the national rules, which meant they could be claimed by anyone who passed the means test, without any kind of assessment of need. This rule applied to all independent homes, not just those run by voluntary organisations and charities. The result was a rapid explosion throughout the 1980s in the number of independent residential care and nursing homes. Numbers and costs virtually doubled each year, fed by rising demand for services in a time of recession and property boom and bust. As biographer of the welfare state Nick Timmins put it, 'unwittingly, the Conservatives had created a new state-financed, if privately run, industry' (Timmins, 2017). A further social security benefit, the residential care allowance, could be claimed by people in independently run care homes but not local authority or NHS establishments. This was another incentive for the NHS to accelerate its withdrawal from long-term care and transfer patients into privately run nursing homes. In turn, many local authorities moved quickly to transfer some or all of their care homes to independent bodies whose residents could claim this allowance. It also meant that cash-strapped local authorities avoided heavy building costs for improving and upgrading older buildings that no longer met new registration standards. It should be borne in mind that local authority budgets were and still are, cash-limited, whereas the national social security budget was not. By 1998, local authorities' share of the care home market had plunged to 22 per cent, from 66 per cent in 1975. Conversely, the private and voluntary sector share had shot up from 34 to 78 per cent over the same period. It was a similar story for home care services (LaingBuisson, 1998). The end result is that today, over 90 per cent of social care services are provided by a range of private and voluntary organisations.

It has been impossible to find any evidence of an explicit policy decision that in effect stimulated the creation of a big private market in social care. On the contrary, it seems a classic example of unintended consequences, and so there was no discussion or debate about the implications of relying so heavily on private provision of an essential public service. There was independent regulation to monitor the standards of care offered, but until 2014 no oversight of the risks of business and financial failure. In that sense, care homes were treated no differently from any other business. And the spirit of the times was to favour privatisation, deregulation and the use of market disciplines as a means of improving public services. It took the collapse many years later of a major care provider, Southern Cross, with 31,000 places, to expose the absence of any plans or procedures to anticipate and manage the consequences of market failure on such a scale.

These two major, and linked, changes – the withdrawal of the NHS from long-term care and the shift towards the private provision of public social care – illustrate how some of the biggest changes in social care in our lifetimes have slipped through quietly, unannounced and unplanned, untouched by the endless procession of plans and strategies. A third change is the growth in material prosperity, which follows.

'You've never had it so good'

Wider changes in society since the end of the Second World War have also had profound implications for social care. England has become a wealthier country, enjoying a standard of living and material prosperity that would have been unrecognisable except for the most well off in the 1940s, when life for many was grim. The war had wiped out over a quarter of the country's wealth and the economy faced a balance of payments crisis, a worldwide scarcity of food (still rationed in the UK until 1954) and a growing shortage of fuel. In many towns and cities, bombing had destroyed or made uninhabitable much of the housing stock. We were a nation of renters. Just 33 per cent of people owned their own homes.

By the end of the 1950s, standards of living had improved dramatically thanks to a global economic boom, prompting Prime Minister Harold Macmillan to declare in 1959, "Let us be frank about it – most of our people have never had it so good." The mood of the time was captured in J.K. Galbraith's famous book *The Affluent Society*, but not all boats had risen on this rising tide of prosperity as the 'rediscovery of poverty' in the early 1960s was to reveal (Abel-Smith and Townsend, 1965).

Nevertheless, the scale of the overall transformation was astonishing as Table 2.1 shows. Thanks to high levels of employment and rising wages, the number of people buying

Table 2.1: Changes in personal wealth, 1948–1994 (1990 prices)

Type of wealth	1948 (£b)	1994 (£b)
Net personal wealth (savings, investments and life assurance)	24	705
Housing wealth	10.7	920
Consumer durables	6.7	209
Occupational pension wealth	1.3	743
Private pension wealth	0	140

Source: Blake and Orszag (1999)

their own homes reached 66 per cent by 1994, their ranks swollen further by council-house tenants who took advantage of big subsidies to buy their homes under Mrs Thatcher's right-to-buy legislation. The goal of a 'property-owning democracy' embodied the post-war aspiration for a better future in which home ownership was common across society rather than a preserve of a wealthy view. A boom in house prices in the 1970s and again in the 1980s gave a further boost to housing wealth. The other dramatic uplift in personal wealth stemmed from a doubling in the number of people joining and contributing to occupational pension schemes.

That is not to say the economy has not been without its troubles, the most recent (before coronavirus) being the global recession from 2008, which ushered in an era of falling house prices, rising unemployment and fiscal austerity. Despite the downturn, recent levels of personal wealth are unprecedented. By 2018, the total wealth of private households had reached £14.6 trillion, consisting mostly of pensions (£6 trillion) and property (£5 trillion) (ONS, 2019a). Since 2006–08, savings and investments alone had increased by more than 60 per cent in real terms. Pension wealth has seen the largest overall rise in value. The measured value of defined benefit pensions rose by 75 per cent between 2006–08 and 2016–18, while defined contribution pension pots almost doubled over the same period. It is not easy to relate the idea of trillions of pounds to the numbers we are used to in everyday life. One comparison is that £14.6 trillion is over seven times the UK's gross domestic product (a measure of the size of the economy). It would repay the national debt seven times over.

How this wealth is distributed is far from equal. The richest 10 per cent of families hold around half of total net wealth, while the poorest tenth has negative net wealth: their debts exceed what they own. The gap between these poorer and richer households has widened in recent years (Bangham and Leslie, 2020). It is not surprising that much of this wealth is concentrated in older age groups, as they have had time to save, contribute to pension schemes and pay off their mortgages. When I began my social work career in the late 1970s, the default assumption was that almost all pensioners were poor. That over half of over-65 households now have wealth of £500,000 or more (25 per cent have at least £1 million) is a reflection of the remarkable turnaround in the financial fortunes of large numbers of older people.

But while large-scale 'pensioner poverty' has been vanquished, there are still many older households with relatively low wealth and a significant number are asset rich but cash poor. Despite the much-vaunted triple lock on state pension, which has helped improve the value of the UK's state pension a bit, it is still stingy compared with our European neighbours. There are big differences in wealth *within* as well as *between* generations.

Since these figures were collated, COVID-19 has caused the most severe economic contraction in more than 100 years and will make a dent in this wealth. One assessment suggests that the impact will be greatest on those with low levels of income and wealth (Bangham and Leslie, 2020). People born in the 1960s onwards are accumulating wealth at a much slower rate than their predecessors (D'Arcy and Gardiner, 2017), but the overall level of personal and household wealth will remain high and has big implications for how social care is funded. The figures destroy any notion that, as a country, we cannot afford to spend more on social care. One fruit of our material prosperity is that we can, if we so choose, invest more in a decently funded system of care and support. It seems utterly illogical to deprive ourselves of such a prize on the spurious grounds of unaffordability. The tricky bit of course is how we access that wealth and how much of the costs of care come from the public purse (via taxation of one kind or another) and/or from private savings and assets. These are intrinsically political choices and subject to competing values about the respective responsibilities of individuals and the state.

This success story of financial prosperity and private wealth, unimaginable to the architects of the means-testing regime in 1948, means that the majority of older people of all ages are likely to have assets that easily exceed the current thresholds and will be expected to meet the full costs of residential care themselves. The default position of the current funding model is that the costs of care will increasingly fall on the shoulders of individuals, especially as the means-test thresholds for residential care have not been updated since 2010 (currently at £23,250 in England, £28,000 in Scotland and a munificent £50,000 in Wales). For most younger people (between 18 and 64) the position is different in that most will have been unable to acquire much personal wealth and will be eligible for council-funded care.

The scale of property wealth – £5 trillion – helps to explain why the question of 'selling your home to pay for care' has become such a totem in the politics of social care reform. The home has come to be seen as a personal asset that must be protected from care charges, a view that has garnered strong support in focus groups and deliberative events with the public. Housing wealth has become a big issue and obstacle to social care reform. A better question might be how can people use the wealth that is tied up in their home to have a better life in their later years? There is a much bigger agenda for housing that is less about protecting its value from care charges and more about improving its quality. Homes that are warm, well-insulated and appropriately designed and located will reduce the need for social care and, in many cases, health care.

The key point here is that the extent of our personal wealth does create options and choices for how we pay for care. These will be considered in more detail in Chapter 8.

How many false dawns?

At various points in the last 70 years, politicians and policy-makers have acknowledged that these sweeping social, economic and demographic shifts and advances in medicine, science and technology have together raised big questions about our social care system. Each of the last five decades has seen the government of the day introduce major reforms, all in response to what was seen as the problem of the day.

The 1970s saw the first serious official attempt to create a modern social care function that reflected the changing times. Throughout the 1950s and 1960s, the welfare services for older and disabled people bequeathed by the 1948 National Assistance Act had grown. New psychotropic drugs and plans to close the asylums (of Enoch Powell 'water towers' speech) had given rise to the new concept of community care reflected in the 1959 Mental Health Act. There was growing concern about juvenile delinquency and the need to better support families instead of taking children into care. None of this was helped by the fragmentation of responsibilities between different council departments, not to mention the NHS. As it was observed at the time:

> A good many jokes and cautionary tales were being told about families who were being visited by half a dozen or more social workers ... a family might have dealings with representatives of the children's department, the health department the welfare department and with social workers attached to the housing and welfare departments, all under the same local authority. ... the family which found itself so unable to cope with the complexity and stresses of modern life that it required all these services was the very family upon which the additional burden of coordinating them and of sorting out the possibly conflicting advice should have not been thrust. (Watkin, 1974)

Frederick Seebohm, then chairman of Barclays Bank, was appointed by the government to lead a review of how services should be organised (thus setting a precedent to be emulated by many other governments of appointing bankers, economists and businessmen to carry out independent reviews of social care).

His central proposal was a single unified social services department in every local authority providing a 'community based and family oriented service, which will be available to all. This new department will ... reach far beyond the discovery and rescue of social casualties; it will enable the greatest possible number of individuals to act reciprocally, giving and receiving service for the well-being of the whole community' (Committee on Local Authority and Allied Personal Social Services, 1968). The resulting legislation – the Local Authority and Allied Personal Social Services Act – was passed on the same day as the Chronically Sick and Disabled Person Act, a private member's bill that created new rights and entitlements for disabled people that went far beyond the very narrow provisions of the 1948 National Assistance Act.

The new nomenclature of 'the local authority personal social services' at the time represented, symbolically at least, a great leap out of the shadows of the Poor Law into the sunlit uplands of a universal, comprehensive service. The big new local authority departments became much more powerful than their fragmented predecessors and their expanded responsibilities (including new duties towards children and families) saw several years of big budget increases. As one director of social services at the time, Tom White, recalled: "I don't think there was any area (of activity) in Coventry in those first ten years that we did not get a 15 to 20 per cent increase in our budget" (R. Jones, 2020). He went on to note that Conservative health Secretary Keith Joseph "secured real increases in spending on social services of 10 per cent, each year he was Secretary of State – a previously unheard-of period of sustained growth in social services spending."

Ten years on, the Barclay review of social work (now consolidated into a single generic profession) commissioned by the new Conservative government, reinforced the Seebohm vision by promoting community social work (Barclay, 1982). Looking back, this was perhaps the brightest of all the false dawns that have characterised the public-policy response to the growing importance of social care. It brought together massive organisational change and consolidation, modern legislation based on a progressive, universalist vision for care and support and a period of big spending increases of which we have never seen the like since. Although the organisational landscape looked very different after 1971 and the status of personal social services was raised, in local government at least, the changes did not deliver their promise. It was largely a structural and administrative response to post-war changes, while the 1948 National Assistance Act remained on the statute book as the cornerstone of social care law, and, by leaving the means-testing regime intact, it did nothing to bring entitlement to social care on the same footing as for the NHS, relying instead on new structures for joint planning with the NHS. A huge reorganisation of local government and the NHS in 1974 did not help.

As the 1970s wore on, the financial tap was finally turned off when an economic crisis led to sweeping cuts in public spending. "The party is over," local government minister Anthony Crosland was to warn councils in 1975. The green shoots of a more universal approach to social care were not to survive a cold fiscal climate. From 1978 to 1986, growth in spending slowed right down to an average 2.4 per cent year-on-year, which suggests that even at the height of draconian public spending cuts, the personal social services were afforded more protection than in our more recent decade of austerity (Webb and Wistow, 1987).

The next decade was to see another set of big reforms, but this time triggered by money pressures. By the mid-1980s, social security spending on residential care, discussed earlier, was now out of control and creating financial incentives for people to enter care homes instead of getting the help they needed at home. An incisive analysis by the Audit Commission (now long defunct) led to the government setting up another review, led this time by Sir Roy Griffiths, managing director of Sainsburys and said to be Mrs Thatcher's favourite businessman – 'a grocer helping a grocer's daughter', in the words of one biographer. The resulting report famously described community care as 'a poor relation: everybody's distant relative but no-one's baby', a description that remains apt today (Griffiths, 1988). His view, a controversial one, was that national social security spending should be transferred to local authorities, and they, not the NHS, would have the lead responsibility for social care. Local councils would become enablers rather than direct providers of care. Many were to split their social services staff into 'purchasers' and 'providers', similar to that introduced in the NHS earlier in the 1980s. Social workers were to become care managers, carrying out 'needs-led' assessments instead of people having to fit in with whatever traditional services were available. Their care managers would commission 'packages of care' from private and voluntary providers – a mixed economy of care. After much agonising (local government largely controlled by Labour councils was not well-regarded by a Conservative central government),

Griffiths' proposals were eventually accepted and embodied in the 1990 NHS and Community Care Act. Implementation of the key changes, however, was postponed until 1993 when a bigger political row emerged about the poll tax. To make sure that existing services were not undermined, councils were required to spend at least 85 per cent of the transferred social security money on private and voluntary providers. At the same time, new national standards for care homes, such as minimum room sizes, presented a hefty upgrading bill, which councils with limited access to capital were unable to afford. Many were to close or transfer their homes to private bodies, as discussed earlier.

These changes were momentous. They cemented the central role of the market in the provision of social care – a direction accidently begun by social security decisions some years before, with now a completely different role for councils as commissioners or purchasers rather than providers of care. It was almost certainly the biggest single act of devolution, of money and responsibilities, to local government in modern history and ran against the tide of increasing centralisation of powers in the Westminster government, with the significant exception of devolution to Wales and Scotland. It was driven by a desire not just to control public spending on residential care, but to create better incentives for people to get care at home and offer more flexibility than traditional care provided by councils. Promoting independence and choice was an explicit objective of the reforms, which were generally welcomed and enjoyed cross-party support.

At the time, I was the lead officer for implementing the reforms in a council in the West Midlands. In trying to explain to a local newspaper reporter what practical difference the changes would make to people in the borough, I was to learn an early lesson in working with the media. I offered the example of an older person who might opt to have his favourite meal delivered from his nearby pub instead of the limited fare offered by the meals-on-wheels service. An hour-long interview was reduced to a short piece with the headline 'Wheeling out the bar meals'. The brave new world of needs-led community care was thus reduced to the prospect of 'pensioners getting chicken and chips delivered from their local pub' (Figure 2.1).

Councils were to do a remarkably effective job of bringing spending back under control, bearing in mind that their budgets, unlike that of the Department of Social Security, were not cash limited. With demand rising faster than budgets, some critics

Figure 2.1: Wheeling out the bar meals

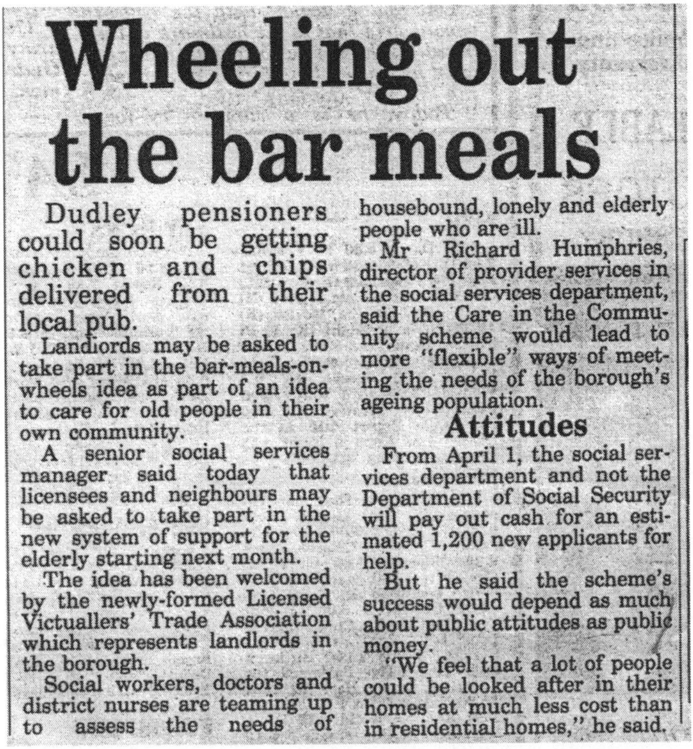

Wheeling out the bar meals

Dudley pensioners could soon be getting chicken and chips delivered from their local pub.

Landlords may be asked to take part in the bar-meals-on-wheels idea as part of an idea to care for old people in their own community.

A senior social services manager said today that licensees and neighbours may be asked to take part in the new system of support for the elderly starting next month.

The idea has been welcomed by the newly-formed Licensed Victuallers' Trade Association which represents landlords in the borough.

Social workers, doctors and district nurses are teaming up to assess the needs of housebound, lonely and elderly people who are ill.

Mr Richard Humphries, director of provider services in the social services department, said the Care in the Community scheme would lead to more "flexible" ways of meeting the needs of the borough's ageing population.

Attitudes

From April 1, the social services department and not the Department of Social Security will pay out cash for an estimated 1,200 new applicants for help.

But he said the scheme's success would depend as much about public attitudes as public money.

"We feel that a lot of people could be looked after in their homes at much less cost than in residential homes," he said.

Source: *Wolverhampton Express and Star*, 18 March 1993

were to describe the transfer of money as a 'poisoned chalice' for local government.

Many of today's problems can be traced back to these changes. One element of the thinking behind the community care reforms was that help should be focused on those with the greatest needs, through assessment and the application of eligibility criteria to determine who received the services. A practical consequence was that traditional local authority home care services gradually ceased to offer a wide range of help, include housework and shopping, and focused instead on personal care (dressing, bathing, getting in and out of bed and so on). It also led to the introduction of checklist-based assessments, arguably at the expense of professional social work judgements, and the greater use of care coordinator and assessor posts that were not necessarily filled by qualified social workers. With it came a new vocabulary of care management, care packages, purchasers and providers, which has not aged well. It was the era of 'the new public management' – the application of private-sector management thinking to public services. For aspiring young managers, the seminal book *In Search of Excellence* by management consultants Tom Peters and Robert Waterman had become influential and *de rigeur* (Peters and Waterman, 1982).

But, in retrospect, no one had thought through what would happen if councils became too reliant on private providers and what would happen if a big provider failed. No one appeared to foresee that the so-called mixed economy was to become much less mixed as the private and voluntary sector market share rose rapidly to over 90 per cent. So much for the original aim of 'promoting a flourishing independent sector alongside high-quality public services' (Department of Health, 1989). The assumption seemed to be that, as long as councils kept 'purchasing' from them, everything would be fine. But, with the dawning realisation that the social security money transferred to councils wasn't enough to meet rising needs, many began to respond to by rationing care instead of empowering their care managers to find creative solutions to individual needs, and, later on, by squeezing the fees they paid to independent providers. Despite the lip service paid to private sector virtues, there seemed little evidence of consumer sovereignty when it came to options and choices for people who used social care. These changes, like those of the Seebohm reorganisation, were to be criticised for not paying enough attention to the voice of people who drew on social care. Whereas Seebohm had tried to put social care on a more universal footing, the effect of the community care reforms threw that direction into reverse. It was to lead eventually to fewer, not more, people getting help, with priority given to people with the highest and most acute needs. Like the Seebohm reorganisation, but for different reasons, the changes proved to be another false dawn, albeit in some respects well-intentioned, in the search for a better system of social care.

An entirely different and more hopeful force for change from a completely different direction had begun a decade earlier, led not by national politicians or policy-makers but by younger disabled people who were unhappy with traditional institutional services and inspired by disability movements in the USA. An early pioneer was John Evans, who lived in a Leonard Cheshire care home in Hampshire. With some fellow residents he established 'Project 81' (a group that rock musician Ian Dury was to call the 'escape committee'):

> Our thinking was this: why should the local authority carrying on paying the residential home? Instead they should transfer the money into an individual's bank account so we could control our own budget and pay our own personal assistants. We negotiated a financial agreement ... which led to us moving out of the institution and living independently in the community. (Evans, 2003)

Thus began the independent living movement and strenuous campaigning to remove the legal obstacles that stood in the way of local authorities making direct payments to disabled people. There were two features of this new approach, which contrasted sharply with the traditional service-led approach: it was intended to transfer power to the individual, so they had more choice and control over their care and support arrangements; and it rested not on assumptions of dependency and deficit but the rights of people to lead independent and meaningful lives in the community, with the same range of opportunities as non-disabled people. They wanted a life not a service. Eventually the Direct Payments Act was passed in 1996. This was later to lead to the policy of personal budgets and offered the promise of a radically different and better way of organising social care. Despite their popularity and cost-effectiveness, however, uptake of direct payments proved to be painfully slow. It was an early example of the apparent inability of the social care system to successfully implement proven innovations so they become available to everyone.

Towards a new century

Although there have been further policy changes since the 1990s which can be loosely described under the headings of modernisation, personalisation and transformation, these grand words were not enough to bring about fundamental change in the way in which social care works.

The incoming Labour government in 1997 recognised that the community care reforms had not worked as intended and their response, the White Paper 'Modernising Social Care', was really about making the existing system work better, not introducing a new one. Its wording reflected the changing political times and the New Labour mantra of 'what matters is what works':

> The last Government's devotion to privatisation of care provision put dogma before users' interests and threatened a fragmentation of vital services. But it is also true that the near-monopoly local authority provision that used to be a feature of social care led to a 'one size fits all' approach where users were expected to accommodate themselves to the services that existed. Our third way for social care moves the focus away from who provides the care, and places it firmly on the quality of services experienced by, and outcomes achieved for, individuals and their carers and families. (Department of Health, 1998)

Here was a new emphasis on closer integration with the NHS, on evidence-based policy-making (of which the creation of the Social Care Institute of Excellence was a practical expression), on driving up performance and quality through a new independent regulator of providers – the new General Social Care Council – and performance assessment – the 'star ratings' of councils. A royal commission was appointed to look at funding, but its central recommendation of free personal care was rejected (this will be considered further in the next chapter).

Meanwhile, the identity of adult social care was to be sharpened by a policy development in a different part of the Whitehall jungle. Since their creation in 1971, local authority social services departments were responsible for the social care needs of the whole population, not only adults. Following a public inquiry into the murder of eight-year-old Victoria Climbie in 2000, The 'Every Child Matters' Green Paper in 2003 proposed a more integrated approach to children's services across social care, education and other services. The ensuing 2004 Children Act required every upper-tier local authority to create a new post of Director of Children's Services responsible for children's social care as well as education and school services. In most places, this meant that the Social Services Department by default became the Adult Social Services Department. By this time, many councils had streamlined their top teams, so that the director of adult social care was often responsible for a range of other council services.

This first decade of the new century witnessed a blizzard of initiatives, plans and strategies covering dementia, learning disabilities and carers. It was a time of high hopes under the reforming zeal of the New Labour government. In 2007, it introduced what it described as 'a major transformation of adult social care' in the ministerial concordat 'Putting People First' (HM Government, 2007). On the face of it, this offered a radical prospectus for change. It commanded wide support – all the main players in the social care sector and six government departments were signatories – and made the bold claim to be 'the first public service reform programme which is co-produced, co-developed, co-evaluated and recognises that real change will only be achieved through the participation of users and carers at every stage' (HM Government, 2007). People would be able to choose their own support through personal budgets, helped by a universal information, advice and advocacy service. A common assessment framework would help iron out variations in what people received depending on where they lived. A new operating model would comprise:

- a shift to prevention and early intervention, to promote wellbeing and independence;
- access to universal information and advice;
- a new model of self-directed support, driven by self-assessment and person-centred planning;
- personal budgets for all entitled to publicly funded care, so people could choose their own care and support;
- a leadership role for councils and their directors of adult social services to achieve whole system change with partner organisations;
- a fundamentally different operating model from traditional services that is based on personalisation (a reformulation of the aims of the community care reforms in the 1990s that services should be moulded to the needs of the individual instead of the other way round).

At this point, the next general election was only three years away. Many of the ideas in 'Putting People First', particularly prevention and personalisation, were echoed in the vision for adult social care published by the incoming Conservative/Liberal Democrat coalition government in 2010 which urged a return to the Seebohm idea of enabling individuals 'to act reciprocally, giving and receiving service for the well-being of the whole community' (Department of Health, 2010). These were all noble aims but, like the Seebohm reorganisation in the 1970s, were soon to collide with another economic crisis.

Follow the money

Until the late 2000s, local authority personal social services – increasingly referred to as adult social care – did well financially. Between 1994 and 2009, they enjoyed more than 15 years of real-term growth, and net spending nearly doubled between 1994 and 2009, an average annual increase of 5.1 per cent. But these percentages began from a relatively small baseline, and the NHS did much better, boosted by the NHS Plan launched in 2000 and Prime Minister Blair's commitment to match EU levels of spending on health care. Much of the increase in social care spend was to cover costs that would previously have been covered by central government through social security payments for care homes so could not be seen as new money as such. In addition, the year-on-year growth was lumpy, ranging from 10.6 per cent in 2002 to a small reduction of 0.3 per cent in 2007–08 and a much lower real growth over the four years from 2005–06. This made efficient planning difficult. Moreover, the extra spend was not keeping pace with rising demand and the strains were beginning to show. Councils were beginning to ratchet up eligibility criteria. By 2012, 87 per cent were limiting help to those with 'substantial' or 'critical' needs, compared with 47 per cent in 2005. The numbers receiving help, especially help at home, began to fall, despite a growing population.

From 2007, there was fresh interest in addressing these financial challenges, but the global financial crisis in 2008 loomed. The writing was on the wall. The Labour government's budget the following year envisaged that total public spending would rise by less than 1 per cent. This translated to a cut in real terms (adjusted for inflation) because of growth in the population and in demand. For social care, it was to get much worse. 2010 ushered in a new coalition government and the beginning of a decade of austerity aimed at restoring public finances. The NHS was to receive a degree of protection from cuts: it had small real-terms increases, but these fell far short of the higher costs of treatment and increased demand. For social care, it was even worse: spending by councils fell by 10 per cent in real terms between 2009–10 and 2014–15 even though most councils had tried to shield social care from cuts (Phillips and Simpson, 2019). Extra money was put in from 2016 – much if it via higher council tax – but hardly enough to make up for earlier cuts. The decade ended with spending barely above 2010 levels (NHS Digital, 2020a).

One ray of hope was the passing of the Care Act in 2014. This had come about from a review by the Law Commission, initiated by the previous government in 2008. The existing patchwork quilt of legislation had been described at various times by judges as 'piecemeal ... numerous', 'exceptionally tortuous', 'labyrinthine' and as including some of the 'worst drafted subordinate legislation ever encountered' (Law Commission, 2011). The 1948 National Assistance Act that aimed to 'eliminate the Poor Law' was to be finally swept away and replaced with a single modern statute.

Legislative reality, at least, appeared to be catching up with policy rhetoric. The new Act sought to recast the duties of councils away from policing eligibility towards promoting wellbeing as the basis of assessing people's needs. It set a new national minimum threshold for entitlement to care and support. There were new duties to monitor and shape the market, in effect playing catch-up with the outsourcing of most care services to independent providers, described earlier. No wonder the Act was widely acclaimed. But, like so many reforms before it, it was implemented in the middle of a raging financial storm such that its high aspirations were seriously compromised by the steepest cuts in council budgets since the 1970s. Part 2 of the Act (discussed in more detail in the next chapter) would have been a milestone in accepting that the state had a bigger role in meeting the costs of care. It was later to be scrapped.

If the Care Act was a ray of hope, the other significant piece of legislation of that time, the 2012 Health and Social Care Act, was not. Popularised as the Lansley reforms (after their architect, health Secretary at the time, Andrew Lansley) it triggered a reorganisation of the NHS famously described as 'so big you could see it from space' (Timmins, 2012). Though concerned mainly with the structures of the NHS, one result was the creation of local health and wellbeing boards, with the aim of promoting the integration of health and social care. The overall effect of the reforms, however, was to make the entire health and social care system even more complex than ever. Then Prime Minister David Cameron was later to rue giving so much time and attention to NHS reorganisation instead of social care reform (Cameron, 2019).

Plus ça change, plus c'est la même chose

This chapter has set out how our lives have been transformed in so many ways since the origins of welfare services in the 1940s, generally for the better. For most of us, our lives are longer, wealthier and generally healthier. Compared with the coupons and queues of the 1940s and 1950s, our standard of living and material lifestyle has changed beyond all recognition. It is worth watching the late Swedish statistician Hans Rosling's memorable and enthralling TED talk to dispel any lingering myths about 'the good old days' (Rosling, 2014). Science and technology have created new possibilities; luxuries have become affordable and commonplace; and our worlds have expanded through travel. Most pensioners are no longer poor. Disabled children are living longer, as are disabled adults. More of us have long-term health conditions that we can live with rather than die from. This is not to gloss over the glaring, and widening, inequalities in how these benefits are distributed across groups of people and places. A consequence of our social and economic success, however, is that most of us at some point in our lives will need some degree of care and support. A growing minority of us will need a very substantial amount of care.

Most governments since 1945, especially since the 1970s, have recognised the challenges in how society offers care and support to its citizens. There have been innumerable reviews, reorganisations, plans and strategies in response to whatever was perceived as the problem of the day. Indeed, this chapter has provided no more than an overview of the bigger initiatives.

There have been many improvements. The protection of disabled and older people from abuse and neglect is rightly regarded as a duty of the state – a relatively recent development since the 1980s. The emphasis of policy, if not always practice, is now placed on the wellbeing of the person using a service and the outcomes achieved, instead of just providing a service. We have come to realise how much traditional service models underestimated the capacity of older people to recover from illness or hospitalisation and recuperate at home instead of entering long-term residential care; likewise, the potential for people with learning disabilities to live in their own homes and hold down jobs, with the right support. The quality of most services is now overseen by an independent regulator, the Care Quality Commission.

But too many aspects of social care have been left untouched by four decades of apparent change. For someone with substantial care needs today, the kind of service they are likely to be offered has changed little since the 1950s. The offer remains home care, day care or residential care, and different approaches and innovations remain small scale. Having emptied the institutions in the 1970s and 1980s, we have re-created modern equivalents, in the guise of assessment and treatment units, and filled them with people with learning disabilities. Set against the expansion of needs, hopes and expectations described in this chapter, it is astonishing that fewer people get help with care and support than a decade ago. Changes in the way the numbers were counted in 2015 make comparisons difficult, but, in 2007, nearly 2 million people used social care funded by councils. In 2019, just 838,000 people received long-term care, and, adding in those getting short-term help, the total barely exceeds a million. Instead of becoming a more universal and widely available service, like the NHS, social care is not rising to meet the challenges but arguably retreating into the past. If Nye Bevan were alive today, 'serene' would hardly be the adjective he would use to describe social care.

Andrew Cozens, in his inaugural speech as newly elected President of ADASS in 2003 eloquently captured the dark shadows that the Poor Law continued to cast, with its attendant language of rationing, eligibility criteria, and means testing to sort out the deserving from the undeserving:

> If there had been an 1834 social services conference, it would have been discussing the Poor Law Amendment Act. The big controversy then was the Government telling parishes they had to reorganise themselves into new unions, and stop helping destitute people in their homes. This meant that those seeking assistance had to enter a workhouse. This policy *could* be judged a brilliant success. Within 5 years an estimated 350 union workhouses were

built – many still standing. People here today would argue that councils that are not implementing direct payments or are capping the amount they will pay for care at home are still, basically, following this Poor Law approach. (Cozens, 2003)

One obvious conclusion from these waves of reform is that we know what does *not* work: reorganisations, additional resources, new policy and legislation, assessing council performance, inspecting services. Each might be necessary, but none is sufficient on its own. Another conclusion is that the unintended consequences of policy decisions, not least on social security and the NHS, along with the winds of social and economic change, have trumped formal government policy-making in shaping what the system has become and how it operates.

Chapter 4 will examine the deeper lessons that need to be learned in forging a better social care system that is fit for the future. But first, it is important to understand in more detail how social care works today, what it does, how much it costs and how it fits with other key public services.

3

Understanding social care

"When I use a word," Humpty Dumpty said, in rather a scornful tone, "it means just what I choose it to mean – neither more nor less."

"The question is," said Alice, "whether you can make words mean so many different things."

"The question is," said Humpty Dumpty, "which is to be master – that's all."

Lewis Carroll, Through the Looking Glass

What is it?

It is surprising that, despite all the attention social care has received in the media and by policy-makers, it is hard to pin down a clear definition of what the term actually means (Smith et al, 2019). In 2007, Dame Denise Platt, an experienced and high-profile social care leader in local and national government, was asked by ministers to review how the status of social care could be raised. Her very first conclusion was that the term 'social care' is not well understood by the public and other opinion formers:

> There is no universally agreed definition of the term 'social care' either within the service or beyond. The

term social care is not recognised internationally; it is more common to find reference to personal social services. The term was created to provide a generic label for the people who worked in residential care and other social services who were not social workers. However, there is better understanding and definition of the term 'social worker', which has an agreed international definition. The title 'social worker' is now protected in law. (Platt, 2007)

The NHS website talks about 'social care and support' which it describes as 'services to help you if you need practical support because of illness or disability; or care for someone receiving social care and support.' It goes on to list different types of social care: 'help at home from a paid carer; meals on wheels; having your home adapted; equipment and household gadgets; personal alarms and home security systems so you can call for help (for instance, if you have a fall) different types of housing, such as sheltered housing and care homes' (NHS, 2021).

Much of the discussion has viewed social care as synonymous with personal care, as illustrated by the Royal Commission on Long-term care in 1999: 'Personal care would cover all direct care related to: personal toilet ... eating and drinking ... managing urinary and bowel functions ... managing problems associated with mobility ... management of prescribed treatment ... behaviour management and ensuring personal safety' (Sutherland, 1999).

The report went on to observe that such a definition 'could be regarded as on the tight side. It would, for example, exclude costs attributable to: cleaning and housework; laundry; shopping services; specialist transport services; sitting services when the purpose is company or companionship.'

What social care is was a central question posed by the Law Commission when it began its review in 2008 of the law covering social care. After all, how could it make recommendations about new legislation without being clear about the purpose of social care in the first place? But, as the commission acknowledged, its role was not to set policy but to reform the law and this is reflected in the definition it went on to adopt:

> Social care means the care and support provided by local social services authorities pursuant to their responsibilities towards adults who need extra support. This includes older people, people with learning disabilities, physically disabled people, people with mental health problems, drug and alcohol misusers and carers. Adult social care services include the provision by local authorities and others of traditional services such as care homes, day centres, equipment and adaptations, meals and home care. It can also extend to a range of so-called non-traditional services – such as gym membership, art therapy, life coaching, personal assistants, emotional support, and classes or courses. Adult social care also includes services that are provided to carers – such as help with travel expenses, respite care, and career advice. Finally, adult social care also includes the mechanisms for delivering services, such as assessment, personal budgets and direct payments. (Law Commission, 2011)

All these examples show how easy it is to slip into a view of social care through the lens of services rather than the needs that services are supposed to meet. Many younger disabled people and increasing numbers of older people, are dissatisfied with traditional services like care homes and day centres and want support that is personalised around their particular needs and preferences, not a 'one size fits all' service solution. In response to these concerns, much more emphasis has been placed, at least in theory, on people being given greater choice and control over how their needs are met. Throughout the 2000s, social care was increasingly viewed in much broader terms and was gradually displaced by the term 'care and support' in the hope this would be better understood. By 2012, the coalition government floated ideas for reform based on a definition noteworthy for its use of plain English and the role of social care in giving people opportunities to live their lives:

> Care and support enables people to do the everyday things that most of us take for granted: things like getting out of bed, dressed and into work; cooking

meals; caring for our families; and being part of our communities. It might include emotional support at a time of difficulty or stress, or helping people who are caring for a family member or friend. It can mean support from community groups and networks: for example, giving others a lift to a social event. It might also include state-funded support, such as information and advice, support for carers, housing support, disability benefits and adult social care. (HM Government, 2012)

Although the Care Act that followed did not produce a crisp, clear definition of social care, the statutory guidance accompanying the Act did recognise that 'the core purpose of adult care and support is to help people to achieve the outcomes that matter to them in their life' (outcomes are mentioned 237 times in the guidance) (DHSC, 2022). The promotion of wellbeing from now on was intended to be the guiding principle for local authorities in assessing whether someone has eligible care needs.

These are definitions of social care viewed through the prism of officialdom. What do people who use social care think it is? In 2018, a new grassroots social movement, #SocialCareFuture, began to emerge. These were people exercised by the gap between the rhetoric of the Care Act – all the talk of outcomes and wellbeing – and the reality for people with care and support needs. They have produced a vision of social care that has a totally different starting point from that of conventional services and from the reductionist focus on, as Anna Severwright put it, being 'fed, cleaned and watered':

> We all want to live in the place we call home, be with the people and things that we love and do the things that matter to us, in communities where we all care about and support each other.
>
> If we, or those close to us, have a health condition or disability during our lives, we might sometimes need some extra support to achieve this. This is the role of social care.

> When designed well, social care helps to weave together the web of relationships and support that we all need to lead the lives we want to, with meaning, purpose and a sense of belonging. Together the web of relationships and support that we all need to lead the lives we want to, with meaning, purpose and a sense of belonging. (Crowther, 2020)

This set of ambitions is about as far as you can get from the reality of how social care is perceived by the public, as street interviews carried out by the Frameworks Institute showed:

> The definition of social care was hazy. Most gave vague answers, often using the terms 'social' and 'care' as crutches in their definitions. When discussing what social care involves and who receives social care, respondents mainly spoke in generalities (often talking about 'vulnerable' people) or mentioned a single group of social care recipients (most often, the elderly). Social care was seen to meet basic needs like ensuring that people have enough healthy food, are clean, and are safe from accidents. It was seen as being for helpless people, described in well-intentioned yet marginalising terms. (Social Care Future, 2019)

The nebulous nature of social care makes it easier for it to be portrayed by the media in negative terms. This is not helped by dystopian stories from care homes during the coronavirus crisis, and a relentless focus on the costs rather than the benefits of care: something that threatens our wealth rather than adds to our wellbeing. Most people unfamiliar with social care tend to view it through in what the philosopher John Rawls described as a 'veil of ignorance' (Rawls, 1971).

Few of us have much, if any, awareness of our chances of needing care, what it would be like or how much it would cost. And when social care is seen as a cost rather than an investment bringing benefits, it makes it much harder for politicians to argue for more spending on social care and for raising taxes to pay for it. Low levels of public awareness of social care have been one reason why all governments have struggled to reform social care. In one survey, most people thought that the NHS provided social care, and nearly half thought it was free at the point of need (Shrimpton et al, 2017). It has not helped that different voices within the social care sector do not always agree on what the purpose of social care should be. Public attitudes will be explored in more detail in Chapter 4.

It is tempting, but unwise, to regard a discussion about exactly what we mean by 'social care' as a matter of semantics. Without a clear understanding of what social care is and what is for, it is impossible to describe and design a system of social care that works for people. And without that clarity, it is equally impossible to galvanise political and public support for change, a challenge that will be discussed more fully in Chapter 7.

Who gets care and why?

Another route to understanding social care is by looking at who gets it, where and why. Figure 3.1 shows how many people received long-term care in 2019 – defined as 'any ongoing service or support provided by a local authority to a person to maintain quality of life' – and where they received it. Almost two-thirds were older people, and the majority received care in the community, usually in their own homes. A higher proportion of older people (26 per cent) lived in residential care or nursing homes compared with 18–64-year-olds.

Why do people need help? Councils are expected to collect data about people's 'primary reason for support'. These are listed in Table 3.1, along with some examples, how the need might be seen by the person needing help and the percentage who get social care for that reason, by age group.

A standout feature of these figures is that nearly a half of people aged 18 to 64 using social care do so because of a learning disability. This reflects the improvements in life expectancy and medical advances discussed in the previous chapter. It helps to explain why for some time council directors of adult social services have been reporting this as the fastest rising area of financial pressure.

Figure 3.1: Who gets long-term care?

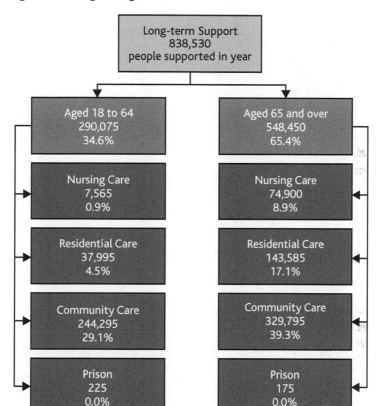

Source: NHS Digital (2020a)

It is less surprising that nearly three-quarters of older people need help with physical and personal care given an anticipated decline in our functional abilities and impact of health conditions, especially in late old age. While personal care – being 'fed, cleaned and watered' – is not the be-all and end-all of modern social care, for most older people, and over a quarter of younger people, it is the main reason why they need support.

There are two provisos to these figures. First, people's lives and needs cannot be neatly compartmentalised into single 'primary reasons'. There is often a lot of overlap between the range of needs, so these numbers give us a broad canvas rather than a

Table 3.1: Why people use social care – primary reasons for support

Primary reason for support	Examples of what this might cover	Why I need support	Percentage receiving long-term care for this reason	
			18–64 years	65 years and over
Physical	Access, mobility such as getting in and out of bed, personal care (help with eating, drinking, toileting, dressing etc.)	"There are physical things I find difficult to do on my own."	29	73
Sensory	Visual impairment, hearing impairment, or both e.g. rehabilitation, skills training, adaptations, mobility and safer travel	"There are things I can't see/hear well enough on my own."	1	2
Memory and cognition	Dementia and cognitive impairment	"My memory or understanding makes it difficult for me to do certain things on my own."	2	14
Learning disability	Help to keep safe from harm or neglect, support to live independently, support with social and educational activities, help with communication	"I find it difficult to learn how to do new things on my own."	47	3

Table 3.1: Why people use social care – primary reasons for support (continued)

Primary reason for support	Examples of what this might cover	Why I need support	Percentage receiving long-term care for this reason	
			18–64 years	65 years and over
Mental health	Support to live independently, go out, have someone to confide in and help stay motivated	"My psychological/emotional state makes it difficult for me to do certain things on my own."	19	6
Social	Support for carers Substance misuse Asylum seeker support Support for social isolation/other	"I am a carer and need support." "I am experiencing substance misuse issues and require support." "I am seeking asylum and require access to support intended for people in my situation." "My situation causes me to be socially isolated."	3	2

Source: Based on NHS Digital (2019)

detailed picture. The second is that these figures relate only to people who are eligible for help through their local council.

A tale of two systems

Most of the facts and figures in this chapter are about people who receive care and support arranged and paid for by their council. But there is a large group of people who pay for their own care and support with their own money because they are not entitled to publicly funded care. This is either because their needs are not high enough to meet the criteria, or their income, savings and assets exceed the means-test thresholds. Very little is known about them, their needs, numbers and circumstances.

The government acknowledges there is an 'evidence gap' (DHSC, 2021a). This is the other system of social care, below the radar of official statistics and largely hidden from public view. The most recent estimate suggests that around 37 per cent of care home residents in England – around 144,000 people – fund their own care, varying from 45 per cent in the South East to 24 per cent in the North East (ONS, 2021). It is not surprising that levels of self-funding are much higher in areas where people are generally better-off and that older people are much more likely to be self-funders than younger people who have had less time or opportunity to save money or buy a house. Knowledge about how many people purchase their own home care is even hazier. The best, but by no means certain, estimate suggests around 230,000 (Henwood et al, 2020). As many self-funders will eventually use up their savings, they will turn to their local council for support. The Care Act 2014 placed a duty on councils to offer advice, information and assessment to everyone, irrespective of their means. However, most councils know very little about self-funders in the area – who they are, what kind of care they are buying and how much they are paying. If self-funders make poor choices without the benefit of advice, often a 'distress purchase' at a time of crisis, they are likely to burn through their money at a much faster rate and seek public funding much sooner. Social care must be one of the few markets where private money can produce both worse outcomes and higher costs.

For the few, not the many

When the numbers of people receiving council-funded social care are compared with England's general population, it is striking that they are so low. In 2019, just 2 per cent of the adult population received long-term and short-term social care. For older people, it is higher: 7 per cent of the over-65s get social care, compared with just 1 per cent of those who are 18 to 64. This is a far cry from the universal reach of the NHS, where getting on for 90 per cent of us use our GP services every year. The population is growing and ageing, with chronic health conditions and disability increasing, so NHS activity is going up, but the numbers receiving social care are heading in a different direction. In every year since 2015 (when there was a change in the way the figures were counted), fewer older people have received long-term care. For 18–64-year-olds, there has been a slight increase. There is now a well-established trend that began in the mid 2000s for fewer people to get social care even though more people are asking for it (Bottery and Ward, 2021). By September 2020, as the coronavirus pandemic continued, the numbers getting long-term help had fallen even further (NHS Digital, 2020b).

There are different possible reasons for this fall. Either councils are cutting their coat according to their cloth and offering less help to people, or they are getting better at responding to needs in different ways so that the need for long-term help is prevented. At least some of the fall will be due to more people not being entitled to public funding and paying for their care using their own savings or assets. The data is not good enough to know exactly how much of the declining use can be explained by each of these possible reasons. Also, the relationship between ageing and the need for social care is not straightforward. The proportion of people age 85 and older with a social care need fell from 49 per cent in 2006 to 43 per cent in 2018, counterbalancing the impact of higher numbers overall (Raymond et al, 2021).

The point here is to avoid making an automatic assumption that fewer people using social care is always and for everyone a bad thing. For some it may be an improvement. We now know that, in the past, too many older people were moved into long-term residential care, particularly when they were ready to be discharged from hospital. This was based on flawed assessments of their needs based on what they could not do rather than what they could if given the right help. For many people, direct discharge into a care home is the least appropriate and most expensive option. Since the 2000s, much more emphasis is placed on supporting people to regain independence and return home through intermediate care (halfway services that bridge the gap between home and hospital) and reablement (short-term intensive help for reacquiring skills after hospitalisation and illness).

It is not just older people for whom these approaches are beneficial. People with learning disabilities, such as Robert (Box 3.1), have been given help to live independently instead of being in a hospital or care home or reliant on traditional day centres. Many places have developed a 'progression model' in which the individual is supported at their own pace to achieve their aspirations by gradually developing their skills and confidence (Bolton, 2016). There is a very strong argument that for most people the first and foremost purpose of good social care is to help people not need it, other than for short periods.

Box 3.1: Robert

Robert is a 26-year-old with a moderate learning disability and autistic traits. He attended residential college for three years before returning to live with family for a short period. Despite using high levels of respite and other support this broke down and led to a period in hospital. He moved to a new service for supporting four people in accommodation where each person has an apartment with their 'own front door'. The apartments are on a single site and staff and others have the ability to respond to crisis where needed. A progression approach has helped Robert become more independent and his support costs have fallen from £3486 to £2003 per week. [This is over three times what councils would normally pay for care for an older person, and helps to explain why many say that learning disabilities services are the fastest growing area of pressure on their care budgets.] (Local Government Association, 2016)

Trying to capture the significance of these different approaches is one reason why the data definitions were revamped in 2015 to distinguish between long-term care, which is likely to be continuous and ongoing, and 'short-term care to maximise independence', which, abbreviated to ST-Max, sounds like a sports drink or a fuel additive rather than a form of social care. ST-Max refers to time-limited support, for example help to get people back on their feet on returning home from hospital, and is intended to reduce or eliminate the need for ongoing support. This is better for the individual and less costly. It is part of a wider approach, described as 'asset-based' or 'strengths-based' practice, that looks to build up people's strengths (Social Care Institute for Excellence, 2018). Such approaches often involve drawing on 'community capacity' in the form of friends, neighbours, voluntary and community groups. There is growing evidence about how councils can improve outcomes for people and reduce costs by drawing on these different approaches to optimising care delivery (County Council Network and Newton, 2021).

Can you help me please?

Understanding social care involves considering the needs and circumstances not only of those who get help but taking a step back and looking at the much larger number of people – 1.3 million – who approached their local council for help with social care in 2019–20. This number has been steadily rising in the last few years (Table 3.2).

These figures hardly suggest that councils are being lavish. Over half of people applying did not go on to receive council-funded support other than that loosely described as 'universal' services. This usually means being given advice or information or put in touch with a voluntary organisation or other support outside statutory services. For many people, that will be entirely appropriate, for there is a world of difference between a routine enquiry or request for information and, for example, a hard-pressed family carer who has reached the end of their tether and desperately needs support. But, as there is no follow-up of people who did not get support, we simply do not know whether the response was appropriate or not. Certainly it seems odd that,

Table 3.2: What happens after people ask for social care

What people are offered	All ages percentage	18–64 years percentage	65 years and over percentage
Universal services or signposted to other services	28	32	26
No services provided	27	35	24
Short-term care	18	11	20
Ongoing low-level support	15	14	16
Long-term care – community	7	6	7
Long-term care – care home	2	0.4	2
Other	3	2	0

Source: NHS Digital SALT reference tables 2019–20, Table 9

whereas requests from 18–64-year-olds have been rising by 10 per cent over the last 10 years, reflecting growing needs and demography, those from older people having been falling. The reason for this disparity is not clear, but it is yet another reminder that social care is about people of all ages.

A final observation. A visiting Martian could easily conclude from media coverage alone that the biggest problem in social care (after people having to sell their homes to pay for it) is hospitals full of older people who are stuck there waiting for a 'package' of social care so they can be safely discharged home. In fact, most of the requests for help received by councils are from people living in their own homes, with just 20 per cent of requests involving people in hospital (NHS Digital, 2020a). This offers a salutary reminder that most of the work of social care, especially at this point of first contact, is about supporting people who are living in their own homes.

This is not to deny the problems of 'delayed transfers of care' from hospitals, both for the patients affected and those waiting to be admitted. It is a particular problem in the UK because we have fewer acute hospital beds per head of population than most other comparable countries. This means that even a small percentage of delays can result in big problems for hospitals operating at very high levels of occupancy. The evidence, however, is that the majority of delays – 60 per cent in 2019–20 – are down to issues within the NHS rather than social care (NHS England, 2020). Social care does far more than just help the NHS clear hospital beds, and, by working with primary care and community health partners, can play a vital role in helping people avoid hospital in the first place. However, cuts in local authority social care spending have led to significant increases in the number of older people attending the emergency department, especially the oldest and those living in the most economically deprived places (Crawford et al, 2021).

The money maze

A different angle again to understanding social care is to 'follow the money' and look at what is spent in England and where that money comes from. In 2019–20, the government spent around £540 billion on public services of all kinds in England (HM Treasury, 2021). In the same year, local authorities spent £19.7 billion on adult social care – just under 4 per cent of the total (NHS Digital, 2020a). In these terms, compared with the big beasts of social protection (mostly pensions) and the NHS, social care is a fiscal minnow.

The money that councils spend comes from a complicated mix of sources shown in Figure 3.2. Unlike the NHS, there is not a single national settlement whereby the government decides how much money will be spent on social care. Instead, this sits with councillors in each of the 151 councils responsible for social care (depending on where you live, this could be a county council, London borough, unitary council, city or metropolitan borough). Every year, each council considers the relative priorities they should give to social care alongside other services for which they are responsible, such as libraries, children's social care, refuse collection and public health. It will agree how much should be spent on each service and set the level of council tax accordingly, weaving together several strands of money to form an annual budget for the year ahead. It may come as a surprise to discover that only 11 per cent of what councils spend on social care comes from central government (Figure 3.2). Most of this is not ring-fenced, which means

Figure 3.2: What councils spend on social care: where the money comes from

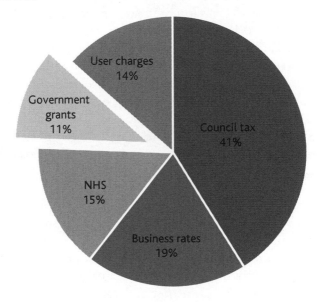

Source: Local Government Association, 2019–21 figures

there is no requirement for councils to spend it on a particular service. Local government has usually supported this, believing that councils are best placed to make decisions about spending priorities based on local needs, not the Westminster government.

Since 2010, the amount of financial support from central government has fallen by 40 per cent in real terms, with government policy increasingly expecting councils to become financially self-sufficient through council tax and business rates. Part of the rationale for this policy was to create incentives for councils to stimulate their local economies to create new jobs and businesses and thereby raise more income. The actual 'spending power' of councils (the total amount they can raise from all sources) fell by an astonishing 29 per cent in real terms over the decade (NAO, 2021a). The upshot is that 41 per cent of council spending on social care now falls on local council-tax-payers, and on local businesses via business rates. This shift has been accelerated by the government's introduction of something called the 'social care precept' in 2015. The precept gives councils the flexibility to increase their council tax by a further percentage to raise more money for social care. In 2020–21, every council levied a precept of up to 2 per cent, which raised almost half a billion pounds. Unlike general council-tax receipts, this amount must be spent on adult social care.

As well as shifting the balance from national to local taxation, a second shift has allowed more care costs to fall on private pockets instead of on the public purse. Charges levied on people who use social care have been slowly creeping up and now account for 13 per cent of council social care spending – that means test again. In comparison, just 1 per cent of NHS spending comes from patient charges, and the rest is raised through national taxation. Some increase in charging has been overt, as when councils have increased their charges for services like home care, day centres and meals. This usually attracts much local opprobrium from the people affected (see, for example, Carter 2021). But much if it has been by stealth. The means-test thresholds have remained unchanged for over a decade, so the effect of inflation sees more people expected to meet at least some of the costs of their care. The means test has got meaner.

There is a particular twist in the privatisation of the costs of care that is even more insidious, and usually invisible to those directly affected by it. Many care homes charge people who self-fund their own care on average 41 per cent more each week than their fellow council-funded residents (Competition and Markets Authority, 2017). They say that this is because the amount councils pay does not reflect the actual cost of care. In effect, this means that self-funders are not only paying their own care bill but also contributing to part of the costs of their publicly funded fellow residents.

A third shift in how social care is paid for is the increasing use of NHS money to support social care, largely through an initiative introduced in 2015 called the Better Care Fund (BCF), worth £3.8 billion. This was not new money as such but drawn mostly from the budgets of local clinical commissioning groups that are responsible for commissioning health services for their local population (Bennett and Humphries, 2014). Originally trumpeted as a flagship policy to integrate social care with the NHS, it required councils and the local NHS to jointly agree how this pooled budget should be used to support social care services. Its backstory offers another example of how differently social care is treated in the allocation of public money. The government's spending review in 2010 – the one that heralded a decade of austerity in public services – protected the NHS budget from real-term cuts, but not local government. The BCF really amounted to the government snipping a small hole in the ring-fence around the NHS budget to help relieve the mounting pressures on social care. The snip was, of course, hedged with bureaucratic reporting requirements to make sure it was spent to benefit the NHS. It has now become a sizeable chunk of money on which councils rely, augmented by an 'improved' BCF from 2015, which saw some of the money given directly to councils as a government grant instead of channelled through the NHS. In 2021, the BCF amounts to £6.7 billion, of which £4 billion is from the NHS (DHSC, 2020b). But, as the NHS England Chief Executive at the time, Simon Stevens, warned, "no one should pretend that just combining two financially leaky buckets will magically create a watertight funding solution" (NHS England, 2014). The NHS also spends a lot of money (£4.5 billion in 2017–18) on paying for people's social care under its responsibility for continuing healthcare (discussed later under 'Who pays').

This is a simplified account of where councils get their money from to pay for social care. It sits within a system of local government finance of byzantine complexity that has eluded the efforts of many governments to simplify and make fairer. The community charge, or poll tax, for example, provoked riots in the streets and helped precipitate the downfall of Margaret Thatcher (Moore, 2019). In 2017–18, the government provided local councils with 250 different grants, half of which were worth £10 million or less nationally (Local Government Association, 2021). This was before the myriad of new grants given during COVID-19.

The complexity of these funding arrangements creates three major problems. The first is that, while councils are accountable to their local electorate for what they spend, the fact that they draw on at least six separate funding streams, three of which are beyond their control, makes it impossible to demonstrate accountability for how much and how well money is spent. This enables the government of the day to say that they have given generously to councils and it is up to each council to decide how much priority they wish to give to social care. In this interpretation, the social care precept is just one more recent tool the government has employed to pass the parcel back to councils. It is equally possible for councils to riposte that the amount in question is inadequate and it is all the fault of the government for not funding councils properly. A further twist in the spiral of blame happens when care providers censure councils for not giving them enough money to meet the true costs of care. So, instead of central government, local government and care providers working together to achieve the best outcomes for people with the money available, a cycle of mutual recrimination and buck-passing is hardwired into the system.

The second problem is that the way the money is raised has become increasingly unfair. Almost 40 per cent comes from council tax, which is based on property values that are 30 years out of date and is highly regressive, falling disproportionately on the less well-off (Adam et al, 2020). The social care precept has made this worse, because councils with the greatest social care needs, usually in places with higher levels of economic deprivation, are not able to raise as much money as better-off areas with a higher council tax base (Smith et al, 2018). In 2020, affluent areas like Surrey, Richmond on Thames and Dorset raised twice as much money per person from the precept than Birmingham, Blackburn and Hartlepool, which have the highest deprivation scores in the country (author's own calculations). Not having a single national funding deal for social care leads to what has often been called the 'postcode lottery' – that the care people are offered depends as much on where they live as it does on what they need. Different councils have different levels of funding and make different decisions about how much to spend and on what. This is not so much a lottery but an inevitable consequence of the convoluted funding system presided over by many governments of all political persuasions.

A third problem is that, although the government has put more resources into adult social care over the last four years, it has done so through short-term, time-limited and one-off injections of cash, which makes it hard for councils to plan ahead and make best of use of the money. This encourages the perpetuation of the status quo, with tight budget settlements only permitting changes at the margins. There have been at least 12 specific and separate funding announcements between 2016 and 2020 (Foster, 2022). The absence of a long-term spending settlement for social care has been a major obstacle to social care reform, and will be discussed in more detail later.

In conclusion, if there was an international prize for the most complex and confusing, least transparent, inefficient and ineffective way of raising money for local services, England would surely be among the frontrunners if not the outright winner.

The social care pound

What councils spend on social care, and where they get the money from, is just part of the jigsaw. It does not tell us the whole story about the much greater sums of public and private money actually spent on all of the activities and costs associated with caring for people.

Starting with private money: as well the charges levied by councils, there is the care privately purchased by individuals who are not entitled to any public funding care, as discussed earlier. These are essentially private transactions between individuals and care providers, so there is no reliable official data. The best estimates suggest this spend could be around £11 billion; not far off half as much again as what councils spend (DHSC, 2021a). Over half of all care home fees are met privately (including payments from relatives to top-up council fee rates). Thirty per cent of people use their own money to buy more care and support over and above what their council pays for (LaingBuisson, 2021). Then there is the work of voluntary organisations in social care supported by fundraising from members of the public – another £4.8 billion (NCVO, 2021). The value of the social care pound could be swelled further if the worth of community assets, such as neighbourliness, volunteering and local associations such as faith groups, could be quantified and included.

Bigger still are chunks of public money allocated through the benefits system administered by the government's Department for Work and Pensions (DWP). In England in 2019–20, £32 billion was paid out in financial benefits to support the additional costs of disability and long-term illness. Granted, not all of these benefits are focused on care needs. The employment and support allowance (ESA), for example, helps to meet the living costs of people with a disability or health condition who cannot work or are trying to return to work. Another £2.7 billion is spent on the 'carer's allowance', equivalent to the princely sum of £67.50 per week. If we adopt a broad view of the purpose of social care, namely, to enable people to live a fulfilled, meaningful life as independently as possible, then all of this is relevant expenditure. A measure of growing need is that the government's own estimate is that it will be spending over 11 per cent more on all of these benefits by 2025 (Department of Work and Pensions, 2020).

What puts all these public spending figures in the shade is the estimated value of unpaid care provided by family members and other friends and relatives. If anything, this increased during COVID-19 and is now estimated to be worth £193 billion a year in England (Carers UK, 2020). It is often not appreciated just how dependent the social care system, and the NHS for that matter, is upon unpaid carers. Were they to go on strike, formal services would be overwhelmed very quickly.

Much of the discussion about the problems of social care revolves around the penurious state of council finances as though this represented the entirety of the system. In reality, the bulk of social care has little to do with officialdom; instead consisting of the quiet and invisible efforts of around 9 million people across the country, in the privacy of ordinary homes, who care for and support a relative or close friend. The position of unpaid carers will be considered further in Chapter 6.

Putting together all these pieces of the funding jigsaw gives us a much bigger picture of the social care pound (Figure 3.3). There is no rhyme or reason to how these separate lumps of public and private money are put together to deliver good care

Figure 3.3: The social care pound

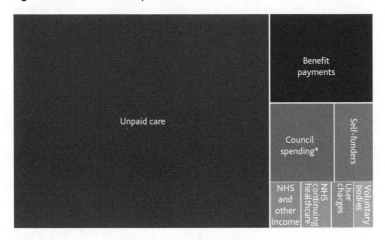

Benefit payments

Unpaid care

Council spending*

Self-funders

NHS and other income

NHS continuing healthcare

User charges

Voluntary bodies

*Council spending adjusted to avoid double-counting income from NHS and user charges

and support. The oft-described problems of joining-up the NHS and social care are but one example of the many fractures in the landscape of public services that run much deeper. Different pots of public money are used by different parts of the welfare state with different rules (unlike council care budgets, DWP benefits such as attendance allowance do not come from a cash-limited budget) and with no shared purpose or coordination. A good example is the relative ease with which I was able to obtain attendance allowance (AA) for both my parents of up to £90 per week to help with care costs, although many will be less equipped than I was to grapple with the 28-page DWP claim form. AA is a benefit that is universally available to anyone aged 65 and over in such circumstances, irrespective of income and wealth – there is no means test.

Much of the debate about social care has overlooked the bigger quantum of public money and private effort expended on social care. The size and scope of the social care pound is such that we could be much more imaginative about how this very large aggregation of public and private resources could be better used to meet people's needs. This in turn could open up new opportunities to consider how we pay for care.

Who pays?

If only the complexity of how social care is funded were just a matter for academic and policy experts. For people who need social care, finding out how much and in what circumstances they have to pay can be daunting. Although there is a national set of rules governing how councils should work out how people have to pay towards their care home costs, based on the means test described earlier, it is by no means simple or straightforward. The official guidance goes into 118 pages of great detail about how different kinds of income, benefits, savings and assets should be treated when carrying out financial assessments. Councils have much more discretion in how they set charges for other services, such as home care, but they must never apply charges that would reduce someone's income below a certain weekly amount: the minimum income guarantee. Some services should not be charged for, such as intermediate care and reablement (free for up to six weeks), assessment and advice, minor aids and adaptations.

Despite the political gnashing of teeth about people having to sell their homes to pay for care, most people with social care needs are not that well-off, especially those of working age who usually are not in paid employment and have had no opportunity to acquire savings, property or pensions. If you are reliant on state benefits, care charges are a very big deal, and concerns have been raised about charges going up during the pandemic (Carter, 2021). Even for care homes where there are prescribed national rules the extent to which people such as Margaret (Box 3.2) are expected to contribute comes as an unpleasant surprise.

Box 3.2: Margaret

Margaret is 83 and is moving into a care home. She lives in a rented flat and has savings of £10,000, which will not be taken into account because it is less than the threshold of £14,250 beyond which she would have to contribute. But her income is a different matter. She has state pension of £125.95 and a further pension credit of £51.15, giving a total weekly income of £177.10. All of this will be taken towards her care home costs, bar the £24.90 she will be left with for personal living expenses. So, in this case, although Margaret is entitled to financial support from her council, she will still be contributing £152.20 per week.

Margaret would like to move to a care home that would be closer for her to children to visit, but this would cost £750 per week. This is £100 more than the council assess is necessary to meet Margaret's needs. Her children agree to pay £100 per week to top-up the council's rate. So, in this case, although Margaret is entitled is council funding, a third of the costs are met by Margaret and her family.

The hit on Margaret's pocket could have been much bigger had she more savings or capital, such as a house. (A reminder: anyone with resources exceeding £23,250 will have to pay their care costs in full. For sums between £14,250 and £23,250, they will contribute on a sliding scale. Only when it drops below that lower amount does the council pick up the bill in full. And even then, they will have to give up most of their income.) For disabled people getting support at home and reliant on benefits, the impact of social care charges on their incomes can be equally dramatic. Despite the minimum income guarantee discussed earlier, councils take into account pensions, means-tested benefits and others including personal independence payment, disability living allowance and attendance allowance in working out how much someone has to pay.

> Take Sarah, aged 34. She has a learning disability and lives in supported housing with social care support for meals, budgeting and running a home. She gets housing benefit for her rent, but with no assets and being unable to work, Sarah is reliant on disability benefits for all other essentials such as food, fuel, council tax, social activities and clothes. She has been paying £81 a week towards her care package but last April the council told her that this would increase to £125. (Hansard, 2022)

But for many, the most glaring anomaly and unfairness of all is whether the NHS or the local council is responsible for paying for their care. People such as Ray (Box 3.3) whose needs arise primarily from health issues, due to disability, illness or accident, can apply for NHS continuing healthcare (CHC). If successful, the NHS will be responsible for providing for all of that person's assessed health and associated social care needs, including accommodation if that is part of the overall need. In the course of a year, around 110,000 people are deemed eligible for CHC, a number that has begun to drop. The costs are significant – around £4.5 billion in 2017–18 – and fall on the budgets of local clinical commissioning groups (CCGs). No wonder in 2019 the government required the NHS to make an 'efficiency' saving of £855 from this budget (House of Commons Library, 2020).

These different funding streams encourage the NHS and councils to push the funding responsibility onto each other, with the person needing care and their family caught in the middle. The legal duties on CCGs to provide CHC are fuzzy. Only 20 per cent of people who apply for CHC receive it. Not surprisingly, the judgement about where the boundary should fall between health care that is free at the point of use and social care that is means tested has been the subject of countless complaints, legal challenges, court judgements, and ombudsman rulings. Many people are not aware of CHC, or have to wait too long to be assessed (sometimes dying before a decision is made), or find the whole process complicated and stressful. There is a twelve-fold variation between CCGs in awarding CHC (House of Commons Committee of Public Accounts, 2018). The financial consequences for individuals can be immense, but the human costs even greater, as Ray's story shows.

Box 3.3: Ray (as told by his daughter Sally-Ann)

My father, Ray, who suffered from dementia, was admitted to hospital with pneumonia 11 weeks before he died. He was already known to social services with a care package in place, so we thought the process for discharging him would be pretty straightforward – how wrong we were! He could not be left unsupervised as he was unable to do anything for himself. He was at risk of malnutrition, dehydration and pressure sores and prone to recurrent infections. None of this seemed to be defined as a health need, and it took five weeks to reach a decision about whether he was entitled to continuing healthcare as health and social care fought over who should pay. Where was the person in all of this? It was decided that he didn't qualify. But then began our next battle. Dad's care package had to be arranged through the hospital's social services team which meant that he could no longer have the care agency he had been using for the previous two years – which had given him the same carer every morning for five days a week. She had become like part of the family. The carer becomes part of your life – the first person you see after a sleepless night and the one who is always there for you day in and day out. For my mum, this was a huge blow. They were taking away the only familiarity and support they both so needed at this time. Mum felt like a stake had been driven through her heart. Her beloved Ray was dying and her carers were being taken away too. Bear in mind that the monthly bill for my dad's care was running into four figures. The community nursing team tried one last attempt at getting continuing healthcare funding for Dad and even 24 hours before he died, they turned him down. A visit once a day to change the pump, and a night sitter for his last three nights was the health-funded contribution. What I now ask is: why should anyone at the end of their life have to pay for their own care to die at home? (Commission on the Future of Health and Social Care in England, 2014)

If this was not complicated enough, there is a further payment available for people in England who are not entitled to CHC but are assessed as needing care from a registered nurse and live in a nursing home. This is called NHS-funded nursing care (FNC). In 2021, this is worth £187.60 per week and is paid directly to the home

The upshot is that the funding of someone living in a care home will be a made up of as many as six different funding sources – from the council, NHS continuing healthcare, NHS-funded nursing care, joint funding by the council and the NHS, means-tested charges from their own money and contributions from relatives. For people who have care at home, there are different issues about the interaction between care charges and benefit entitlements, and these raise a different kind of complexity.

Not free at the point of use

Not only is social care worlds apart from being free at the point of use like the NHS, the horribly complex way it is funded is a recipe for conflict between those seeking help and the public bodies charged with providing it. If coming up with a better way of funding local services has defeated the sharpest minds of Whitehall and academia, then imagine what this means for people who need social care. Seventeen per cent of social care complaints to the local government ombudsman in 2020–21 were about charging and, of these, 72 per cent were upheld (Local Government and Social Care Ombudsman, 2021).

It is not just the money aspects that make social care so difficult for people to understand and navigate. Figure 3.4 visualises just how bewilderingly difficult it is, showing the multiple ways in which an individual could potentially access care in England. Add in the severe financial pressures that assault councils and care providers, it is no wonder that many people like Chris (Box 3.4) use words like 'struggle', 'battle' or 'fight' to get the support they or their relative needs.

Box 3.4: Chris

I had to fight to get the best for my mum. I threatened to go to my MP and the director of adult social care. You've got to find out as much as you can, and dig and dig and dig. Nobody is going to do it for you. There is a range of benefits that everybody is entitled to. I wasn't aware of any of this at the start. I am now! (Which? 2021)

Figure 3.4 punches home how social care has lost sight of its primary purpose of supporting people to live the best life they can. Instead, it has to come to resemble a bureaucratic steeplechase, with twin hurdles to jump to demonstrate that you are poor enough and needy enough to be eligible for very basic help. Bryony Shannon, who works in social care, offers an apt description:

Figure 3.4: Funding routes for adult social care in England: care pathway model

Residential care

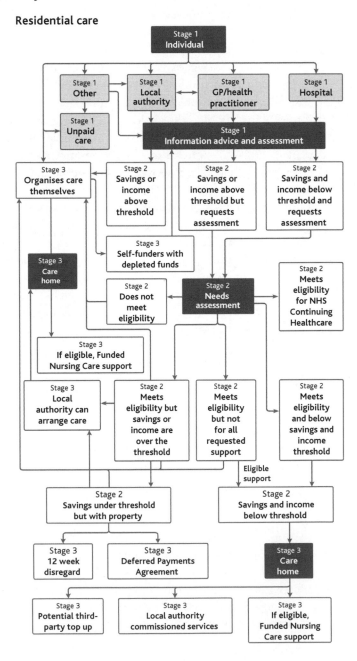

Community care

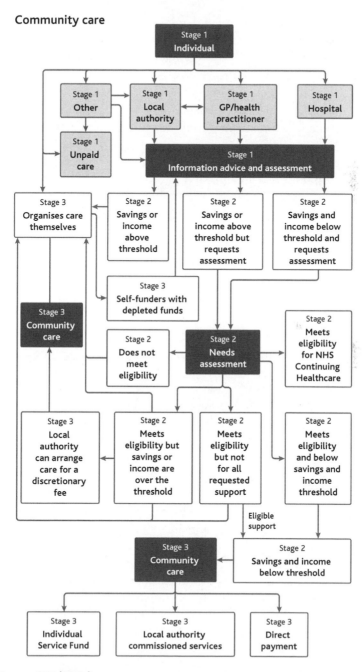

Source: ONS (2021a)

Often by the time we meet you, you've been screened. Triaged. Discharged to assess.

We've identified you as vulnerable. At risk. In need. You've ticked the right boxes.

You've become a referral. An allocation. A concern. A case. We've read details about your problems and your conditions and your needs from forms. Our records reflect your life through the lens of (usually multiple) 'professionals'. We're already forming an impression of you, possibly already determining your (our) outcome.

The majority will be your four calls a day stuff.

Our assessments and reviews allow us a snapshot of you, a glimpse in an intense, pressurised situation. You – or people close to you – answer pre-determined questions about what's wrong and what you can't do. You're under pressure to say the right thing, without being totally sure what the right thing is. To score enough points to proceed.

If we identify you as 'eligible', we plan and provide services to maintain your existence, to keep you alive, then close your case and move on.

If we decide you're 'not eligible', we signpost you elsewhere, then close your case and move on. (Shannon, 2021)

The complexity and arbitrariness of the system is described by Jonathan, a retired civil servant, who describes a 'catalogue of errors' in getting the right care for his mother, Gillian, who had dementia and needed residential care:

Despite being modest schoolteachers, my parents had saved up to make sure that they could look after themselves and their family moving forward. I could see that by renting her house out, one month of rent would cover less than one week of care home fees. If you had the equivalent of a village thermometer for the new church steeple, you could see the thermometer working its way down through her savings quite rapidly. I could see where we were going, so we applied for funded nursing care and continuing healthcare. You would not believe how much nagging and delays we had. Finally, the nurse assessor came. We all sat round the room. We did an assessment at the end of which, probably wrongly, she said, 'Yes, you're right, she should get funded nursing care. We are really sorry for all the delays. I'll recommend that it be backdated.' I thought, 'Great.' That meant that she would still be contributing. Her pensions and other income would still contribute to her care costs, but that extra bit of pretty modest support would mean that her house and any savings would be protected from that point moving forward. That seemed to me like a pretty reasonable deal. I should say that my brother, who lives abroad, when mum first went into a care home, said, 'Ah well, of course, that will be paid for by the state.' I just laughed. I was pretty aware of the broader situation. It was a very hollow laugh. There has never been an argument that there should not be some support that we should pay for, and that mum should pay for from her money. Six months later I said, 'Is the benefit coming through? I haven't seen it yet.' The care home was still charging the same amount. I had been warned that it could take a long time. It turned out that the assessor had never filed the paperwork. She had registered it on the computer system but had never filed the paperwork. They said, 'Don't worry, we will get that in.' What they neglected to say was that they had then decided to do a peer review, and took a decision – having never met my mum and having never been part of the assessment – that actually she did not qualify and, terribly sorry, there were no funds coming. The way in which they handled that was appalling. They would not tell me the reasons. They did not even tell me there was that panel, so when I appealed because I thought it was an admin mistake, it transpired that it was not. It was an utter catalogue of errors. We were back in the same position, with my mum's hard-won savings being used to fund her care. (Health and Social Care Committee, 2021a)

Gillian's condition deteriorated and another application for continuing healthcare was submitted, but after more delays, this too was turned down. An appeal was submitted, but rejected two months before her death. When asked what would have made a difference, it is not difficult to find scores of stories like this, featuring words such as 'Kafkaesque', 'bruising', 'harrowing', 'appalling'. Jonathan was asked, 'What would have made a difference in enabling your mother getting the care she needed?' His reply: 'A much more understanding and accessible system and for it to be much more transparent about what support is available. I had to find out so much of this.'

In 2018, I was involved with Ipsos Mori in some deliberative work with members of the public to find out what they thought of social care and how it should be funded. Two day-long workshops were held in three different locations in England: London, Leeds and King's Lynn, attended by 116 people. I was struck that, although most people taking little part knew little about social care, those that had experienced it were in many ways none the wiser. They found it frustrating trying to find a way through the bureaucracy to access help and knowing who to contact. Some thought their GP would be the first point of contact. Few mentioned councils unless prompted. In the words of one participant: "The biggest thing I found is no one seems to know where to get help. Not knowing where to go, or who to get advice from, to get everything started. There doesn't seem to be any one place." And another: "I've had to try to use it, but no one really wants to give you the full ins and outs of what you're entitled to and what they can do and when they can do it" (Ipsos Mori, 2018).

A matter of opinion

What do people who use social care, and the wider public, think? NatCen Social Research's British Social Attitudes (BSA) survey is widely regarded as the gold standard for surveys of public views about a variety of social topics including attitudes towards health and social care. Usually, public satisfaction with social care is low – 29 per cent in 2019, a figure that has not changed much in recent years. This compares to 60 per cent for the NHS, a seven-point jump on the previous year. The top reasons people gave for this rating were the quality of NHS care (68 per cent), the fact that the NHS is free at the point of use (60 per cent) and that it has a good range of services (49 per cent) (Appleby et al, 2020).

One explanation for the difference might be that, as we have seen, at any one time only a tiny proportion of the general population use social care, compared with the NHS. In 2019, for the first time, the survey tried to measure differences between people who had experienced health and social care compared with those that had not. People who had used social care in the last 12 months were more likely to be satisfied (a conclusion that applied to NHS services too): 38 per cent, compared with 27 per cent among those who had not.[1] But that is still well below satisfaction levels with the NHS. And those who had experienced social care were also more likely to be dissatisfied – 47 per cent – than those than those who had not – 35 per cent. The difference with the NHS is again striking. Dissatisfaction with social care services was high for those both with and without recent contact compared with other health services. The most likely explanation is that those who have used a service tend to have an opinion on satisfaction, one way or the other, while those who have not tend to take a more neutral position (or say they don't know). That a trip to the dentist should elicit twice the satisfaction rating of using social care is cause for reflection.

But is social care really so bad? Most people who use social care apparently think not. Every year, the Department of Health and Social Care commissions through local councils a survey of the views of people who use adult social care. In 2019–20, 64 per cent said they were 'extremely satisfied' or 'very satisfied' with their care and support and a further 24 per cent were 'quite satisfied' (NHS Digital, 2020c). Although these ratings have dipped very slightly over the last five years, it is striking that they are so high given the very well-publicised problems of the sector and the impact of financial austerity on council care budgets over the last decade. At one level, these figures suggest that everyday experiences tell a different story from the national narratives of policy neglect and financial insufficiency. They offer an important reminder of the good that social care can do.

There are, however, some important provisos about these findings and why they should be treated with caution. The DHSC survey does not include people who pay for their own care. One interpretation of these high satisfaction ratings is that the declining numbers of people who actually get into the publicly funded system have a relatively good experience but at the expense of those who fall outside it. The views and experience of the latter are largely unknown. Within the 62,520 people surveyed, there are also some surprising variations. For example, although most people prefer to get care and support in their own home (and most do) they are less satisfied: 57 per cent are extremely or very satisfied, compared with 71 per cent of people in care homes and 63 per cent in nursing homes. Those aged 18 to 64 are more satisfied than older people; white people are more satisfied than their black and ethnic minority counterparts; and Londoners are less satisfied with their care than people in other parts of the country (NHS Digital, 2020c).

In a separate survey, carers report much lower levels of satisfaction. Only 37 per cent were extremely or very satisfied, and 7 per cent were very or extremely dissatisfied – an ominous sign given how much the system depends on them.

Measuring people's attitudes is of course notoriously tricky, especially in situations where people feel dependent on those providing the service and might be reluctant to be critical. Responses can be skewed by all kinds of cognitive bias. People, older people especially, may confuse satisfaction with gratitude and relief, and sometimes are prepared to overlook negative aspects of their experience to avoid rocking the boat. Here is an example cited in one study:

Interviewer: I'd like to ask you to rate how satisfied you are with the services that you had for your husband. So how satisfied from a scale of extremely satisfied … [shows flashcard with Likert scale]

Carer 29 WB: [interrupts] Probably quite satisfied, yes.

Interviewer: So quite satisfied with the carers that came in to help your husband?

Carer 29 WB: Yes.

Interviewer: So why would you say quite satisfied?

Carer 29 WB: Well as I said they had such varied, and some would come in and would speak over my husband, and I had to say, well he's there, he can hear, he knows everything that's going on. You had to sort of stop them speaking ... as if he wasn't there, or treating him just like an object instead of a person. (Willis et al, 2015)

Here's another example from the same study of someone who offered a positive satisfaction rating because she had a really good relationship with her social worker, despite having to wait eight months for support:

SU 31 SA: She [my social worker] was fantastic, so I was extremely satisfied with her, and I felt that she heard me, and I felt that she got through the whole process as quickly and as effortlessly as possible given the situation.

Interviewer: So 'given the situation', do you mean there were constraints?

SU 31 SA: Or should I say given the nature of her workload and the things that I was going through, so really it was a case of us being patient with each other yet having a good communication in between. You know, it took about, it took almost eight months for me to get my support.

In conclusion

This chapter has set out to understand social care through different lenses – of needs, numbers, money and attitudes – and this throws some light on why reforming it has been such a tough nut to crack. The different terms used to describe it since 1948 – welfare services, personal social services, care and support, social care – shows how it remains a slippery concept that means little to most people and lacks the brand recognition of the NHS. It is trying to meet an array of individualised needs that defy a simple definition, covers all ages and everything from end-of-life care to helping younger people lead a good life as independently as possible. Everybody wants different things from it. The spaghetti-like mix of funding sources has obscured just how much the financial burden has shifted insidiously from central government to individuals, families and council-tax-payers. This has created ideal conditions for a blame-game between government, local councils and care providers. Accountability is blurred. It is hard for people to access and navigate social care, and, although more people are asking for help, fewer people are getting it. It is described euphemistically as the social care 'system', implying a designed collection of components that fit together and works. It could be more accurately described as the gradual historical accretion of random, ad hoc acts of policy, shaped by the unintended consequences of developments in other public services, notably the NHS and benefits system, all played out in the different geographies of local places.

Whereas good social care ought to be a unifying feature of a good society, instead, enfeebled by a decade of austerity and years of muddled and short-term policy-making, it has been turned into multiple arenas of conflict. Councils are turned against providers in setting fees; local NHS commissioners and councils try to shunt costs to each other, policing the boundaries and budgets of their services; and people are resorting to the language of military warfare to describe their struggle to get essential support. For too many people, the purpose of adult social care seems to be to keep them out of the system, sometimes camouflaged in the benign language of signposting, resilience and 'asset-' or 'strength-'based practice.

On whose shoulders the financial and human costs of care fall is often a product of random chance not rational policy-making. Yet there is a much bigger 'social care pound' that offers opportunities to think differently about the future. This raises big questions about how different governments have tried to tackle these issues, why they have failed and, crucially, how we can learn from history instead of repeating it.

4

Learning from the past

> Between the idea
> And the reality
> Between the motion
> And the act
> Falls the Shadow
>
> > T.S. Eliot, 'The Hollow Men'

Non, je ne regrette rien?

Danish philosopher Soren Kierkegaard once said that life can only be understood by looking backward; but it must be lived looking forward, an aphorism that is highly germane to understanding past efforts to tackle social care reform. There is no shortage of former ministers, prime ministers, even, who appear to undergo a Damascene conversion about the importance of social care reform once they have left office. David Cameron, prime minister between 2010 and 2016, has written movingly of his family's first-hand experience of the good that social care can do, recounting the support he received with his severely disabled son, Ivan, including carers organised by the council: 'I found the phone number of Kensington and Chelsea council's social workers and soon, to my great relief, one of them was sitting in our kitchen, notepad in hand, talking about the help that was available' (Cameron, 2019). Years later, he was to describe his government's failure to deliver social care reform as 'one of my greatest regrets.' There is no mention of social care in Tony Blair's account of his ten years in Downing Street, nor in his successor's, who seemed more exercised by how to integrate social care with the NHS (Brown, 2017). Norman Lamont, Chancellor of the Exchequer in the 1990s, interviewed by historian Peter Hennessy in his Radio 4 series *Reflections*, was asked, if he could be granted one last reform, what it would be. "Care of the elderly," he replied, describing it as "the great unresolved issue of public policy" (BBC, 2019). More recently, Jeremy Hunt, the longest serving Secretary of State for health and social care, has said that one of his biggest regrets about his time in that role was that social care was not better protected from austerity. 'It was the silent cut that people didn't notice until too late', he said (Sodha, 2021). 'Our social care problem is now critical ... so why the delay in fixing it?' he asked in another newspaper article, admitting that having secured a substantial ten-year funding settlement for the NHS, he failed to do the same for social care. 'I was told it would follow – but it never did' (Hunt, 2021).

It is not as though governments, of all political hues, have not tried. A huge amount of policy-making energy and political debate has been expended on finding solutions to the problems of social care over the last three decades. As noted earlier, since 1997 there have been at least 14 government White Papers, Green Papers and consultations of kind or another. Success has eluded 5 governments, 10 secretaries of state and 15 ministers for care services drawn from three political parties. There have been at least five independent reviews or commissions, two of which were commissioned by the government. Parliamentary select committees have conducted four inquiries in the last two years alone. Unlike many countries across the world, such as Australia, Germany, Japan and the Netherlands, that have managed to implement major reforms, England has continued to struggle to come up with a wide-ranging and sustainable response to what many see as one of the most pressing public policy challenges of our time. Everyone agrees something must be done, but no one can agree what that should be or find a way of seeing it through.

Instead of trudging through the disheartening detail of every attempt, it is worth summarising the key landmarks and how these have played out against the political timeline of the last 25 years. Further detail can be found in a very good timeline on the King's Fund website, the first version of which I helped to prepare in 2014. I had no idea at the time that were would be at least another eight years to go (King's Fund, 2021).

Labour and the National Care Service, 1997 to 2010

Social care funding reform was already on the political agenda when Labour was swept into power by a landslide majority in 1997. The year before, the Conservative government had floated ideas about insurance and pension solutions to care funding in a consultation paper entitled 'A new partnership for care in old age'.

Following Tony Blair's landmark speech saying he didn't want his children to grow up in a country where the only way older people could get care was by selling their home, his new government got off to a flying start in 1997 by fulfilling its manifesto commitment to establishing a royal commission, 'With Respect to Old Age', which reported in 1999. On receipt of the findings, however, the government didn't like the central proposal of separating accommodation and living costs from care costs and making the latter free at the point of use. Even the commissioners did not agree: in a 'note of dissent' to the main report, two of them described free personal care as a 'chimera' that would need a 'Croesian flood' of higher public spending. They argued that this would be unaffordable and, in any case, would largely benefit the heirs of the well-off (Sutherland, 1999). As one of the commissioners was to comment: 'The majority recommended what they thought the Labour Government *should* do. The minority what they thought the Labour Government *would* do' (Timmins, 2017).

Instead, the government introduced some adjustments to the existing system, such as 'free nursing care', through a new allowance for people in nursing homes. Today, this is known as NHS-funded nursing care, discussed in Chapter 2, and is worth £187.60 per week to successful claimants from April 2021. Social care funding then returned to what was to become its customary domicile for much of the next two decades – the so-called long grass. North of the border, the Scottish Executive took a different view and used its new devolved powers to introduce free personal care for older people from 2002. In 2019, it was extended to people under 65 years old.

The underlying concerns about the inadequacy of the current system continued to simmer. The early years of the new century saw significant, if uneven, rises in public spending on social care, but not enough to allay returning fears about the widening gap between the numbers needing care and available resources. By the middle of the decade, spending, on older people in particular, had plateaued and then begun to fall as councils began to ratchet up their eligibility criteria, as discussed in Chapter 2. For the NHS it was, as ever, a different story, with Prime Minister Blair on breakfast TV in 2000 committing to raise NHS spending to the European Union average – later to be dubbed 'the most expensive breakfast in history' (Timmins, 2021). The Treasury asked former banker Derek Wanless to carry out an independent review of NHS spending. His final report in 2002 concluded that health spending and social care spending should be considered together, recommending that a much more detailed assessment should be made of social care's funding needs. This was not acted upon, by the Treasury at any rate. So, the King's Fund commissioned him instead. With substantial input from the LSE, the central recommendation from Wanless's meticulously researched 300-page tome was a partnership funding model that offered everyone a minimum guaranteed level of care, with the state matching private spending pound for pound (Wanless, 2006). Similar thinking was emerging from work by Donald Hirsch at the Joseph Rowntree Foundation, underpinned by the proposition that the public will be more willing to pay more for a system that they perceive to be fairer (Hirsch, 2006). A newly formed 'Caring Choices' coalition of care organisations engaged with more than 700 people at events across England and Scotland and through an interactive website. It called for a much simpler system that offered people a clearer entitlement to care (Caring Choices, 2008).

The combination of policy thinking and campaigning led to funding reform coming back into play, signalled by a fresh commitment in the 2007 Spending Review to 'look at reform options and consult on a way forward.' A new flurry of policy activity and public engagement led to a consultation paper, 'The case for change – Why England needs a new care and support system', published in May 2008 and based on 'a clear vision for care and support that promotes independence, choice and control.' This 'vision' had emerged from an earlier government consultation in 2005 as part of New Labour's public service reform programme – the 'Independence, Well-being and Choice' Green Paper. Interestingly, this stated that 'implementing the vision will need to be managed within the existing funding envelope' (Department of Health, 2005). Having developed the vision, the next step was yet another Green Paper, 'Shaping the Future of Care Together', in July 2009, launching a public consultation called 'The Big Care Debate' (HM Government, 2009). This set out proposals for what was to become Labour's flagship social care policy – a National Care Service that, in the words of Prime Minister Brown, was 'fairer, simpler and affordable for everyone – a service underpinned by national rights and entitlements but also personalised to individual needs, where everyone can get the best possible care whatever their particular circumstances and where carers themselves also receive the support they need' (HM Government, 2009a).

The Green Paper recognised that, to make this vision a reality, difficult choices would be needed about how it should be funded. It sketched out three broad options: a partnership model, such as that proposed by the Wanless review; an insurance approach, involving some costs met by the state and the remainder funded either by private or state-backed insurance; and a 'comprehensive' option under which everyone over the age of 65 would be required to pay into a state insurance scheme. It suggested an indicative range of £17,000 to £20,000 per person, which could be paid by instalment or as a lump sum, before or after retirement or after death. A free care system for people of working age would operate alongside this. The option of funding care entirely through general taxation was rejected on the grounds that this would be place a heavy burden on people of working age.

'The Big Care Debate' was described as the largest ever public consultation on social care, involving 68,000 people through 37 stakeholder events, 80 public roadshows, supplementary qualitative research and direct contributions in writing or via a website. Ending in November 2009, the government moved swiftly to present its formal proposals in March 2010 through the White Paper 'Building the National Care Service'. It described six founding principles of this new service:

1. Prevention and wellbeing services to keep you independent
2. Nationally consistent eligibility criteria for social care enshrined in law
3. A joined-up assessment
4. Information and advice about care and support
5. Personalised care and support, through a personal budget
6. Fair funding, with a collective, shared responsibility for paying for care and support. (HM Government, 2010)

Hailed by its authors as the biggest single change to the welfare state since 1948, it was to be delivered through a staged five-year programme of reform, initially by building on the best of the current system, seeing through the strategies already in place for people with dementia, learning disabilities, carers and personalisation; implementing reablement everywhere and introducing a new policy for free personal care at home for those with the highest needs. The latter came as a surprising and unexpected announcement by the prime minister, halfway through the consultation process, and not mentioned in the Green Paper. The second stage would be to implement clear, national standards and entitlements, though these would continue to be delivered locally by councils. From 2014, care entitlements would be extended so that anyone staying in residential care for more than two years would receive free care after the second year. But, on funding, although the government made clear its preference was for the 'comprehensive' option put forward in the Green Paper, how this would work in practice – and crucially how much would be paid by whom – was fudged:

> At the start of the next Parliament, we will establish a commission to help to reach consensus on the right way of funding the system. The Commission will determine the fairest and most sustainable way for

people to contribute. It will make recommendations to Ministers which, if accepted, will be implemented in the Parliament after next. The Commission will determine the options that should be open to people so that they have choice and flexibility about how to pay their care contribution. (HM Government, 2010)

So, once consensus on funding had been reached, the final stage of reform would see the comprehensive implementation of the National Care Service, to parallel the NHS, 'for all adults in England with an eligible care need, free when they need it, whoever they are, wherever they live and whatever condition leads to their need for care.'

But the government had run out of road. Just one week after the White Paper was published, Prime Minister Brown went to Buckingham Palace to seek the dissolution of Parliament, and the resulting general election was held on 6 May. This meant that most of the discussion about Labour's proposals for a National Care Service was conducted in the heat of a general election campaign. Even before the White Paper had been published, a political row had broken out over allegations that Labour was quietly considering a 10 per cent levy on people's estates to pay for care. The Conservatives, who favoured a voluntary insurance solution, deployed its now infamous 'death tax' election poster – a picture of a tombstone with the inscription 'R.I.P. off – Now Gordon wants £20,000 when you die. Don't vote for Labour's new death tax.'

Cross-party talks between Andy Burnham, then Secretary of State for health, Andrew Lansley, his opposition shadow minister, and Liberal Democrat Norman Lamb that had begun weeks earlier in effort to find common ground, collapsed in acrimony and recrimination (Bentley, 2010).

Coalition government, 2010 to 2015: Dilnot and the Care Act

Whatever the promise of a National Care Service, the immediate prospects for change disappeared along with Labour's 88-seat majority. But the newly formed government was quick to acknowledge the 'urgency' of reforming social care. With strong influence from Liberal Democrats in the coalition, it committed to establish a commission on long-term care, to report within a year. The commission was asked to consider a range of ideas, 'including both a voluntary insurance scheme to protect the assets of those who go into residential care, and a partnership scheme as proposed by Derek Wanless' (no mention of Labour's comprehensive option). The jointly agreed programme for government that contained this pledge also had a portentous footnote signalling the dark shadows of austerity that was about to begin: 'the deficit reduction programme takes precedence over any of the other measures in this agreement' (Cabinet Office, 2010).

Nevertheless, the coalition moved swiftly to establish the Commission on Funding of Care and Support, chaired by the economist Andrew Dilnot. Its report, 'Fairer Care Funding', was published on time in July 2011. The report's central recommendation was to put a 'cap', or maximum limit, on how much individuals would have to pay for their care over their lifetime. It proposed a figure between £25,000 and £50,000 (equivalent to £36,000 and £71,000 in 2023 prices). Alongside this, it proposed raising the upper means-test threshold – below which people would begin to get public funding from their local council – from £23,250 to £100,000. Those entering adulthood already having care needs would be eligible for free state support. This was an important recommendation given the impact of charges on working-age people with care needs discussed in the previous chapter.

The commission's terms of reference were tightly focused on how the costs of care should be shared between individuals and the state, rather than on the bigger question of how social care should be funded and how that money should be raised. It saw social care essentially as an insurance problem. In the absence of financial products like those that enable us to insure our lives and property, how could people be afforded protection from the uninsurable risk of needing a lot of expensive care that would otherwise fall almost wholly on their shoulders? Nevertheless, it made a recommendation that in the light of later events turned out to be prescient: 'The Government should both implement our reforms *and* ensure that there is sufficient, and sustainable, funding for local authorities. Local authorities will need to be able to manage existing pressures as well as the new requirements resulting from our reforms' (Dilnot, 2011, emphasis added).

A further White Paper and a consultation on funding reform led to the government eventually accepting Dilnot's central recommendations, albeit with a higher cap set at £72,000 and a upper means-test threshold of £118,000. Legislation followed with the Care Act 2014. This covered the Dilnot changes and created a new legislative foundation for social care that would sweep away the 1948 National Assistance Act (see Chapter 2). The hope was that, by the state underwriting the very high costs of those at the tail end of the distribution curve, it would incentivise the insurance industry to come up with products that would be viable and attractive to the larger numbers of people with a much lower risk of needing a lot of care. It was an expectation based more on hope than experience (Chapter 5 looks at the use of insurance in other countries). Remarkably, the Treasury even went as far as identifying how the significant costs of the reforms, estimated at almost £6 billion over five years, would be funded. It was through changes to National Insurance and the freezing of inheritance tax thresholds to provide: 'a simple and fair way of ensuring that those with the largest estates, who are more likely to benefit from social care reform, help to fund it' (HM Treasury, 2013). By past standards, this was real progress. But it was to be short-lived.

Conservative government, 2015 to 2021

The Dilnot plans offered a cogent answer to how the costs of care could be shared between the individual and the state in a fairer way, especially for those facing extremely high 'catastrophic costs', namely the one in ten people likely to need at least £100,000 worth of care, a ratio later upgraded to one in seven. Despite Dilnot's warning, there was no plan to address the mounting pressures on local authority social care budgets arising from swingeing cuts in central government grants to councils. The Local Government Association wrote to the government in July 2015 asking that implementation of part two of the Care Act, covering the Dilnot reforms, which was due to be implemented from April the following year, should be delayed; and that the money earmarked for the reforms be put instead into local authority budgets. So it was that just weeks after the 2015 general election, the new Conservative government postponed part two of the Care Act until April 2020. The rationale was summed up by care minister Alistair Burt: 'a time of consolidation is not the right moment to be implementing expensive new commitments such as this, especially when there are no indications the private insurance market will develop as expected' (Department of Health, 2015).

So, the Local Government Association got its wish, but not the money. Not a penny of it was reallocated to support councils, and the Dilnot proposals were eventually to be abandoned altogether. It was back to square one in arguing the case for funding reform. As I blogged at the time:

> 'While the government has set out a clear agenda and £8 billion of new investment for the NHS, its decision leaves it with no plan for social care other than to reconsider the zombie policy of private insurance which has gained no traction despite ministerial efforts to persuade the insurance industry otherwise. Funding reform has gone backwards five years.' (Humphries, 2015)

Although the Dilnot plans enjoyed wide support, this was never universal. Some commentators argued that improving the quality and availability of care for everyone should be a higher priority than protecting the savings and wealth of relatively better-off older people. So it was not altogether surprising that, despite its previous support for the principle of the proposals, the idea of a cap on care costs was repudiated entirely in the Conservatives' 2017 election manifesto because they 'mostly benefited a small number of wealthier people.' Instead it promised 'the first ever proper plan to pay for – and provide – social care' with three proposals it considered to be fairer, across and within, the generations. They were:

- including the value of the family home in the means test for care at home, bringing it into line with the means for residential and nursing home care, 'so that people are looked after in the place that is best for them';
- to introduce a single means-test floor of £100,000 so that people would always retain at least £100,000 of their savings and assets, much more generous than Dilnot's proposal and the existing system;
- the ability to extend the deferred payment scheme for residential care to those receiving care at home, meaning that the cost of care could be reclaimed from the person's estate after their death, so fulfilling the pledge that no one should have to sell their home in their lifetime to pay for care (Conservative and Unionist Party, 2017).

All this was to be paid for in part by means-testing the winter fuel allowance for pensioners and scrapping the triple lock on state pensions. This was controversial given the traditional reluctance of parties to antagonise older people, who are much more likely to vote. The net result was political uproar. The omission of a cap on care costs was seen as reneging on a previous commitment to implement Dilnot. This was not a matter of fuzzy wording or an oversight. Then health Secretary Jeremy Hunt told BBC Radio 4, "Not only are we dropping it [the cap], but we are dropping it ahead of a General Election and we're being completely explicit in our manifesto that we're dropping it" (BBC, 2017). There was a rationale for its omission, explained by an unnamed ally of Theresa May:

> I have a fundamental problem with someone on a low wage driving a bus in the northeast of England, who can never expect to inherit through housing … any significant amount of money contributing through tax to ensure that someone whose house is worth half a million pounds, is able [to pass] that almost intact

as an inheritance for the next generation. And that's
fundamentally wrong. (Elliott, 2021)

Four days later in a screeching U-turn, Theresa May insisted
that 'nothing had changed' and that her promised Green Paper
would after all include an 'absolute limit' – a cap – on how much
people would have to pay. But the greatest ire was aroused by the
plan to include the value of the family home in the means test
for home care – quickly dubbed 'the dementia tax', although
it would not just affect people with dementia (BBC News,
2017). It seems the term was coined not by the Conservatives'
opponents but by a former speech-writer to Michael Gove and
it appeared in the pages of the right-leaning *Spectator* magazine
(Heaven, 2017).

The controversy about social care was widely seen as marking a
turning point in the election campaign. Instead of the anticipated
landslide victory, the Conservatives lost their parliamentary
majority and remained in government only by doing a deal
with the Ulster Unionist Party. In his resignation statement,
Nick Timothy, chief advisor to Theresa May, went on record
as 'regretting' the decision not to include the cap as well as
the floor in the manifesto (Timothy, 2017). Jacob Rees-Mogg
later described it as 'an untested and frankly disastrous policy;
(Lightfoot et al, 2019). For many, this sealed the fate of social
care as a politically toxic issue that would always end in tears; a
re-run of the 'death tax' row in 2010.

By this time, much of the political oxygen in Westminster
was being consumed by the Brexit psychodrama. The new
Green Paper promised by the government was postponed again
and again, not helped by the resignation in December 2017 of
Deputy Prime Minister Damien Green, who had been leading
the work. Responsibility for producing the Green Paper switched
from the Cabinet Office to the Department of Health (now
with 'and Social Care' added to its nameplate even though it
had always been responsible for social care policy) (House of
Commons Library, 2019). The Queen's Speech in June 2017
stated that the newly elected Conservative government would
'work to improve social care and bring forward proposals
for consultation.'

By the time Theresa May resigned in July 2019, the Green Paper had still to make an appearance. In December, it was reported that it would be a casualty of preparations for a no-deal Brexit, with staff already having been diverted from the Department of Health (Elliott et al, 2018). Though denied by then health Secretary, Matt Hancock, a few weeks later care services minister Caroline Dinenage admitted that Brexit 'had taken centre stage' and distracted from the work on social care (Cecil, 2019). The Green Paper still had not appeared by the time Boris Johnson took over as prime minister in July 2019.

A final fix?

The gap between the idea that social care needs big changes and the reality of achieving it continued, despite Boris Johnson's fresh commitment in 2019. Conservative peer and chair of the influential Lords Economic Affairs Committee, Michael Forsyth, memorably likened waiting for the Green Paper to waiting for Billy Bunter's postal order. Then came the coronavirus, with a government minister declaring: "There simply is not the management or political capacity to take on a major generational reform of the entire (social care) industry in the midst of this massive epidemic" (Hansard, 2020).

The government's priorities for the next parliamentary session, set out in the Queen's Speech in May 2021, contained 30 pieces of legislation, including one for the NHS, but just nine words about social care: 'proposals on social care reform will be brought forward' (HM Government, 2021). At long last, the government did bring forward proposals in the final months of 2021. In September, it published 'Build Back Better', which resurrected plans for a cap on care costs, at a higher level of £86,000 and a more generous upper means–test threshold of £100,000, to come into effect from 2023 (HM Government, 2021a). It was to be paid for through a rise in National Insurance rates of 1.25 percentage points. In December, the government went on to set out wider reforms in a White Paper 'People at the Heart of Care' (DHSC, 2021c).

As with the coalition's proposals in 2014, the Conservative government should be given some credit for seeking to place a limit on the liability of individuals for their care costs for the first time since 1948 – a genuine policy milestone – and for the political courage to break a manifesto commitment to raise National Insurance to pay for it, a very big deal for a Conservative government. However, most of the proceeds of the levy will go to support NHS recovery from COVID-19. Little money remains – £1.7 billion over the next three years – to address other aspects of the crisis in social care including low pay, demographic and other cost pressures (Murray, 2021). The government's proposals will be discussed more fully in the final chapter.

Cycles of failure

Adding up the time taken by each of these failed cycles of reform since the mid-1990s, the equivalent of a decade has been spent in talking about doing something, consulting about doing something and planning to do something. The equivalent of another decade has been spent doing nothing, after the road to reform has petered out and ended up in the long grass. The unique achievement of the Conservative government since 2015 is not just the absence of any kind of progress until 2021 but that it has taken us back several years to 2015, when reforms to the treatment of care costs were on the statute book awaiting implementation, before being cancelled. Six years have been spent on an internal debate raging within the government about the pros and cons of a cap on care costs, the same debate that took place ten years earlier. Arguably, the Labour government should have achieved far more. Without the distraction of Brexit and a global pandemic, it had the advantages of plenty of time, a big parliamentary majority and a favourable economic climate – until the 2008 global financial crisis at least.

Looking back at these past travails, it is possible to discern a general pattern usually with four stages. The first is a light-bulb moment, an explicit recognition that 'something must be done' and a strong political commitment to action. Often this is triggered by manifesto commitments or the election of a new government, for example in 1997 and 2010. The cogs of the Whitehall policy machine grind into action – the second stage – sometimes involving the appointment of a commission and eventually resulting in a Green Paper or some other kind of consultation. Reasonable progress would see this followed by a White Paper with formal proposals. If exceptional progress is made, this results in legislation, notably the 2014 Care Act, with actual implementation tantalisingly close. But at some point in this process, the proposals start to unravel – the third stage. This can involve a combination of reasons, such as a failure to reach agreement (Labour's rejection of the royal commission's recommendations in 1999, for example), competing financial pressures, or nervousness about the scale of the imminent changes, exemplified by the abandonment of the Dilnot proposals in 2016. The fourth and final stage is that the issue becomes politically toxic, is categorised as 'too difficult' and is kicked into that fabled long grass, awaiting the next light-bulb moment. Sometimes stage two has been skipped altogether, proceeding directly from a light-bulb moment to policy meltdown. Typically, this occurs during a general election campaign. The most obvious example is the dementia tax debacle in 2017, where the manifesto proposals appeared to be remarkably undeveloped or tested and quickly wilted under the heat of fierce political scrutiny. Although Labour's National Care Service proposals in 2010 were preceded by several years of policy groundwork, they too could not survive the stress-test of intense electioneering and that death tax poster. It is ironic that both major parties have suffered because of the political weaponisation of social care. As one former care minister put it: 'This is a third rail issue, you touch it politically and you get fried. And I think that's the wrong conclusion. It's a dangerous conclusion, but I fear that that is the conclusion that many in political class have reached' (King's Fund, 2017).

Learning the lessons

Whether history will judge Prime Minister Johnson's commitment in 2019 to 'fix the crisis in social care once and for all' as a light-bulb moment or a momentary flicker of short-term attention will depend on the outcome of the proposals in the 'Build Back Better' plan and the White Paper 'People at the Heart of Care'. The jury is likely to be out for some considerable time. Success this time may depend in part on understanding what lay behind all the preceding failures and how they could be avoided in future; learning the lessons from history instead of repeating another failed cycle of attempted reform. The omens are not encouraging. It as though three generations of politicians in power have taken to heart the late Peter Cook's lament, "I have learned from my mistakes, and I am sure I can repeat them exactly." There is a mixture of reasons, some interlinked, why the road to reform adopted by successive governments to tackle social care has ended up as a road to nowhere.

Lesson 1: Ask the right questions

It has never been entirely clear what – if the reform of social care is the answer – what is the question. Derek Wanless got to the heart of the matter in his 2006 review:

> At the heart of the issue should be a debate about what social care will do in the future. How will it help people? What outcomes should it aim to achieve? Who should it help? Once its purpose is understood and specified, important decisions can then be made about the range and type of services, the size and composition of the workforce, the implications for housing, the use of technology to assist people to live with more control, and the extent of preventive action required to avoid or delay need.' (Wanless, 2006)

It is significant that many of the reform initiatives described earlier have been concerned mostly with how social care should be paid for and where the money should come from. Much of the work on developing a new vision for social care has been silent on what resources would be needed to implement it. This has meant that the focus of reform has been on funding and has become almost entirely disconnected from any consideration of what it is that we want to fund. Of all the policy documents over the years, very few have produced comprehensive proposals to the range of problems and challenges in social care, except perhaps for the National Care Service proposals in 2010 (and even they ducked the issue of how it would be paid for). In turn, the concentration on the money issues has too often focused on finding solutions to one very specific part of the funding problem. The Dilnot proposals were a well-crafted response to the question of how the costs should be shared fairly between individuals and the state, especially for people facing very high care costs. The problem was framed as the uninsurability of the financial risks of care. They floundered because the commission's plea was not heeded, namely that, alongside protection from catastrophic costs, there should be adequate funding for local authorities. It simply became untenable for the government to spend £6 billion over five years in relieving the financial burden on people's private resources without having a plan for people who rely on public funding. It remains to be seen whether the same fate will befall the Johnson government's proposals.

Similarly, proposals for voluntary insurance schemes that have popped up intermittently over the years might have some merit for people with assets to protect from care charges. Other ideas have been floated to encourage people with their own resources to plan ahead for future care needs, for example through care ISAs and pensions. Whatever the merit of these ideas – and they might be very helpful to those who are relatively well-off – they are of little help to people with few or no savings or assets to protect. This is vitally important for younger people with care and support needs, most of whom will not have had the opportunity to acquire much in the way of savings or property.

To seriously tackle the range of problems that currently exist in social care, there at least three sets of questions that need to be addressed:

1. What is social care for? What does good care and support look like; and what level and quality of help should we reasonably expect? As well as meeting individual care needs, how should it contribute to wider social and economic wellbeing? These are questions about purpose and entitlement.

2. How should good care and support be provided and by whom? How should social care work with other public services such as the NHS, housing, benefits and criminal justice systems? What about the wider social infrastructure of communities that affect the needs that people have? Who should be accountable for how well social care works in meeting people's needs? These are questions about organisation and delivery.

3. How much would good care and support cost, now and in the future? How should these costs be shared fairly between individuals, families and the state, taking account of the wildly differing financial circumstances within and between generations? How should the state raise the money to pay for publicly funded care? The questions of funding.

A strong argument can be made that there is a fourth set of questions about *who* provides care, both paid and unpaid, and what is the right balance between the responsibilities of families, communities and the state. A glaring area of neglect in much of the debate about social care reform has been the absence of a workforce plan or strategy. These issues will be discussed in Chapter 6.

Lesson 2: Get the timing right

An evident lesson from the general elections of 2010 and 2017 is that, on the one hand, election manifestos can be a good way of galvanising a high level and general commitment to action. The commitments to an independent commission by Labour in 1997 and the Liberal Democrats in 2010 are good examples. On the other hand, general elections are almost always very bad times to float specific proposals, especially if they involve where the money should come from. Electioneering requires political parties to demonstrate how different and better their policies are than their opponents. Even the most credible proposals are vulnerable to attack. So it was that in the 2010 and 2017 election campaigns, Labour and Conservative pledges on social care were swiftly weaponised politically, with informed discussion and debate quickly displaced by poorly understood but emotive slogans like the death tax and dementia tax. There is a clear message for newly elected governments to set out on the road to reform as early as possible in their first term, having determined the route they wish to take.

There is also a lesson here about taking a joined-up view of health and social care. Derek Wanless in his review of NHS spending had made an eloquent plea to look at social care as well, but this was made politically difficult by Labour's earlier misstep with the royal commission, whose recommendations for free personal care had been rejected by England but accepted in Scotland. The timing, for social care, could not have been worse. As former Treasury official Nick Macpherson has recently noted: 'There had been the Royal Commission. Everyone knew it was a problem. Everyone knew it needed to be addressed. But not this year thank you very much, and so it has continued to this very day' (Timmins, 2021). And Ed Balls, advisor at the Treasury at the time: 'We weren't at the time seeking to solve the social care funding issue. This was about the National Health Service. Five years later it would have been different. One could not have done a Wanless report without social care being in at the beginning' (Timmins, 2021).

The Wanless review played a seminal role in helping the NHS secure long-term investment from the government. The opportunity to do the same for social care had been lost. Instead, from the middle of the decade, Labour spent a lot of time on three separate consultations. By the time it had fleshed out its plans for a National Care Service – seen by many as promising, if lacking detail – the economic climate was deteriorating (always bad news for social care funding) and the timing of its White Paper collided with the general election. The reform timetable was hopelessly out of sync with the electoral timetable. In a similar vein, the current Conservative government may come to regret its prevarication and delay from 2017 in producing proposals before Brexit came to dominate politics, and before coronavirus was to expose horribly the perils of all those years of inaction.

Lesson 3: Aim for cross-party cooperation rather than consensus

As we have seen, efforts to reform social care have been scarred by high-profile bust-ups between political parties, almost always at election time, with the issue ending up back in the long grass. It has become almost an article of faith that progress cannot be made without a high degree of consensus among the major political parties. On the face of it, there are compelling reasons for viewing this as an important success factor. If the reform timeline over 20 years shows nothing else, it is surely that no single government can achieve lasting reform on its own. If Labour with time (13 years), money and a big majority could not do it, the chances of success under current political and fiscal circumstances look bleak. Another reason is that the scale of the change required cannot be achieved in a single parliament and, as with pensions, a long-term approach is needed, a point that will be covered further in Lesson 7.

Although the arguments for cross-party consensus are strong, institutional and cultural barriers get in the way. Cross-party talks to reach such a consensus failed in 2010 and again in 2012, for a mixture of reasons. The UK's first-past-the-post voting system of 'winner takes all' is not conducive to pragmatic cross-party deals that are common in many European countries. It is significant that over the last 25 years, most progress with reform was made in the five years of coalition government when the two parties involved had to agree a programme for government that included a specific commitment to sort out social care. This progress was quickly dissipated upon return to one-party government in 2015. But can the coalition's progress really be ascribed to cross-party consensus? Sally Warren, a former colleague at the King's Fund, was a senior Department of Health civil servant involved in the coalition's deliberations about how to respond to the Dilnot Commission's proposals. She offers an interesting insider view on the dynamics of coalition politics:

> During the many twists and turns of the months of 'Will they, won't they?', we started to get a clear sense not that either party desperately wanted to say yes, but that neither wanted to be the one that said no. Quite often we thought all the signals were that one party was lining up to say no, but when the moment came, it didn't. The policy was being kept alive because neither party could be the one to say no to it. The

political consequence of not acting was different if one side of the coalition could clearly position the other as the unfair blocker of a reasonable proposal. (Warren, 2021)

It may be that consensus is overrated. In contrast to political fighting during election campaigns, the rest of the time it is unusual for political parties to fall out about social care policy. Most if not all of the major legislative milestones in the history of social care since 1948 described in Chapter 2 have enjoyed cross-party support – the Seebohm reorganisation in the 1970s, the community care reforms in the 1990s and the Care Act in 2014. It could be argued that there has been too much 'group think' about social care policy, which has meant that developments such as the drift towards the privatisation of care services, or the withdrawal of the NHS from long-term care, slipped under the radar and did not receive the political scrutiny they deserved.

There is no shortage of examples where MPs and peers have united to call for reform. In 2018, over 100 MPs from all parties, including 21 select committee chairs, wrote to the prime minister urging her to set up a parliamentary commission on Health and Social Care (rather than a royal commission, which would take much longer) to look at funding for social care and the NHS in the round and build support for reforms in parliament (UK Parliament, 2018). The cross-party membership of select committees in both Houses of Parliament have had little difficulty in agreeing recommendations on social care reform, funding and workforce in four separate inquiries in as many years. Here, for example is Conservative Lord Forsyth in the 2020 debate on the Queen's Speech:

> Last year, the Economic Affairs Committee, which I do the best I can to chair, was able to reach unanimous agreement on a way forward. Its membership included two former Chancellors of the Exchequer, two former Permanent Secretaries to the Treasury, a former Cabinet Secretary, a distinguished economist of the left, a retired FTSE 100 CEO, a non-executive director of the Bank of England and other highly experienced

> members. If we could find agreement, why can the
> political parties not? (Hansard, 2020)

Sometimes, the lack of consensus can be used an excuse for inaction. Then Secretary of State Matt Hancock cited this is a reason for the repeated postponements in publishing a Green Paper. He wrote to all parliamentarians in March 2020 seeking their ideas about how consensus could be achieved and promising 'structured talks on reform options in May' (House of Commons Library, 2021). The talks have yet to be convened.

In recent years, differences *within* political parties have been a bigger roadblock to reform than differences *between* them, especially when that party is in government and has the responsibility for making decisions. For some time, there were well-publicised differences in Conservative ranks about the priority that should be given to protecting the family home from care charges as opposed to reducing the tax burden on working-age people. These were laid bare by reactions to the 2017 election manifesto debacle and two years later the pro-Conservative *Telegraph* was talking about 'the scale of the divisions at the highest level of Government over its social care policy', differences that appear to have persisted (Swinford, 2019). Prime Minister Johnson was said, correctly as it turned out, to favour a cap on care costs, whereas Matt Hancock had expressed a preference for voluntary insurance options. There were reports that Chancellor Rishi Sunak was unable to sign off a reform package because the Prime Minister would not allow him to increase taxes to pay for it, although a deal was eventually done (Smyth, 2021). The influence of personalities and political leadership should not be overlooked. Some of the biggest annual funding boosts in the history of social care were secured by the unlikely character of Sir Keith Joseph and his negotiating skills and personal commitment as Secretary of State in the 1970s (interview with Robin Wendt, cited in Timmins, 2017).

So, although there is a strong argument for seeking cross-party support for long-term changes – if only to prevent a new government ripping up the plans of its predecessors, as the Conservatives did in 2015 – there is no reason why a government with a large majority should not at least begin the process, providing it can agree with itself about the direction of travel.

In the current febrile political climate, it is hard to see how all parties could agree on some of the very tricky funding choices when there are sharply differing views among the public as well as politicians (these will be discussed shortly). In the short term, it might be that cooperation is a more realistic ambition than consensus – getting agreement to some principles and a process for arriving at a solution, and ideally a suspension of party-political warfare so that each other's ideas can be a given a fair hearing.

Lesson 4: Improve public awareness of social care

Chapter 2 described how social care began in 1948 as a replacement for the Poor Law, offering a safety net rather than a universal service that everyone would use like the NHS. We should not be surprised that it is so poorly understood. Whereas polls consistently show that the NHS in the eyes of the public is a national treasure and the biggest reason to be proud of being British, social care on the other, is, as Roy Griffiths observed in his 1988 review, 'everybody's distant relative but nobody's baby.' Because such a small proportion of the population actually draw on social care at one point in time, most people are generally unaware of the risks that they or close relatives will need social care, how much good care would cost and the extent of their financial liabilities under the current system. Whereas financial planning for retirement is generally seen as important, planning for future care needs is not. Many believe mistakenly that social care is paid for like the NHS. It registers very low on the scale of the public's priorities when asked by pollsters. For many years, Ipsos have conducted a monthly poll in which a representative sample of the public are asked to say, unprompted, what they see as the most important issues facing Britain today. Typically, in recent years the top issues have included Brexit, the NHS, immigration and the economy, with social care rarely mentioned unless it has been a big news story for a number of weeks. The highest score it ever achieved was 18 per cent in June 2017, after the election of that year. Concern was greatest among social grades AB (27 per cent), people aged 55 and over (26 per cent), Conservative party supporters (24 per cent) and women (Ipsos Mori, 2017). It scraped back into the top ten of important issues at 12 per cent in September 2021, but not for long (Ipsos Mori, 2021a). These perceptions, or lack of them, hardly encourage politicians to take social care very seriously compared with weightier correspondence in their inbox. A director of adult social services captured it pithily:

> We are asking government to prioritise something that the vast majority of voters don't understand and/or don't want to think about. And it is not that surprising. Nobody wants to think about diminishing powers as you grow old, and for working age social care you assume it won't happen to you: until it does. (Humphries and Timmins, 2021)

As long as the public view the issue from behind a veil of ignorance, there will be two direct consequences for any government that wants to do something about it. The first is that politicians trade on ignorance and fear when opposing their rivals' proposals, such that slogans like the dementia tax and death tax cut through. This helps to explain why the Conservatives' manifesto proposals in 2017 had such a mauling, and in one respect unfairly so. Their plan to increase the means-test threshold to £100,000 would have represented a four-fold improvement to the existing position. Instead of being applauded for generosity, it was condemned as an outrageous incursion into private savings, with most people unaware of how mean the current means test is. The second consequence, and perhaps the most serious, is that it makes it next to impossible for any government to engage with the public in an open and transparent way on choices about where the money comes from. It is much easier for governments to contemplate raising taxes to pay for better public services when the public support that service and are assured the money will be spent on it. A notable example is Gordon Brown's decision in 2002 to hike National Insurance contributions to raise an extra £40 billion for the NHS. This was, as a former Treasury mandarin observed: 'the only serious, non-forced, discretionary tax rise since at least 1979 – and one that proved electorally appealing' (Timmins, 2021).

The Johnson government is hoping to pull-off something similar by increasing National Insurance to pay for a health and social care levy from 2022, and early polling suggests this might have worked, with 58 per cent of people supporting the move, according to one poll in February 2022 (Buzelli et al 2022). It is a moot point whether this support would have been as high if the NHS had not been the primary beneficiary of the increase.

Raising public awareness about just how mean the current means test is, and the potentially limitless liabilities for care costs, has to be an essential precursor of discussion about how social care is funded. The good news is that it is possible to do this, as well as emphasising the benefits of good care and not just its costs. There are some good examples of how engaging with the public can raise awareness and make it possible to have sensible and evidence-based debate: the 'Big Care Debate' in 2009, deliberative events with the public organised by Ipsos Mori in 2018 and a Citizens Assembly exercise also in 2018 (Involve and House of Commons, 2018). In England the #SocialCareFuture movement is forging new ways of securing public support for better social care by promoting the value, rather than the cost of care, and the rewards that it can have in helping people to lead a good life. More examples can be found further field, such as the 'Every Australian Counts' campaign[1] and 'Caring Across Generations'[2] in the USA. These offer the potential to adopt a different approach to policy-making and will be considered further in Chapter 7.

Lesson 5: Don't begin with the hard stuff

In recent years, and before COVID-19, the issue of social care has hit the headlines in the context of its financial problems. The big political rows have been about the hard choices of where the money should come from. Choices about tax and spending are intensely controversial. The clearest example is the totemic issue of whether people's housing wealth is a legitimate source of care funding and how much of it should come from general taxation instead. With social care, the public is confronted with the prospect of taking a new financial hit, one way or another, for something they are barely aware of, let alone all of the problems with how it is funded currently or the quality and availability of what is on offer. It is like being presented with a bill and having no idea of what it is for, whether you might need it, or what might happen if it doesn't get paid. As George Osborne, Chancellor of the Exchequer from 2010 to 2016, has observed, the political consequence of fixing social care 'is incredibly unpopular. It's much more straightforward politically to keep kicking the can down the road' (Institute for Government, 2021).

This approach has been entirely the wrong way round, with little preceding effort to engage the public (noting Lesson 4) about the nature and scale of the challenge, or asking them what kind of social care system we need in the 21st century. What form might it take? What benefits would it bring and what might it cost? Then, and only then, should debate progress to the options for how it could be funded. This of course underlines the importance in Lesson 1 of asking the right questions about what it is we need to fund. The 'Big Care Debate' in 2009 was an attempt to carry out this essential groundwork. But, as we have seen, the Brown government ran out of time and the debate took a different direction after the 2010 election. As Andrew Dilnot pointed out, echoing George Osborne's point:

> Where there is not consensus is where the money should come from that is what is always politically most toxic for Governments. The debate is much more now about where the money should come from than about what the money should be spent on. My advice for any institution trying to build consensus would be try to focus on that. (Health and Social Care and Housing, Communities and Local Government Committees, 2018)

In a recent interview, former health secretary Andy Burnham's advice to today's reformers is clear: 'Don't start with the money – don't start saying, "We'll stop you spending this" or "We'll protect your home." Start with a vision for what health and care should ideally look like in the 21st century' (Elliott, 2021).

A clear finding from deliberative work with the public is that when they are talked through the issues and understand better the benefits of good social care for themselves and the wider community, they grasp the fact that it will need more money. They accept that raising money to pay for it will not be painless and are up for a debate about the pros and cons of different ways of doing that. However, if politicians in power see social care primarily as a money problem, the Treasury becomes the dominant force in calling the shots and can seek to restrict open discussion, as Sally Warren explains:

> At no stage has government openly talked about where that money could come from, and what might the trade-offs be. Indeed, at every step, government has done whatever it can to avoid that conversation – with HM Treasury asserting that it and it alone decide these things. One of the more infuriating moments in my social care reform journey was being told in response to a popular reform option 'Of course people like it, it's a free lunch' when at every stage in the preceding two years HM Treasury had refused to allow any debate or discussion about how to pay for the increased costs. (Warren, 2021)

Lesson 6: Avoid paralysis by analysis

It is not for want of policy reports, analysis and reviews that social care remains unreformed, with bookshelves groaning under the weight of at least a quarter of a century's worth of outputs from governments, charities, think tanks and academia. A whole range of policy options, involving private and public funding, have been assessed, analysed and quantified. The experience of other countries has also been canvassed in pursuit of the 'right' solution for England. As we have seen, in government, Labour carried out four separate consultations on social care between 1997 and 2009: one on quality, a second on a vision for social care and a further two on funding. Spending so much time on discussion and analysis ran down the clock and barely left any time at all to develop and deliver proposals, much less implement anything substantial. Faced with internal differences and external distractions, it took the Conservative government four years before it got around to publishing its proposals. In summary, over the last 25 years, the machinery of policy-making seems to have lurched backwards and forwards from frenzied overactivity to sleep mode.

Arguably, we have spent too much time considering policy content – the 'what' of social care reform – and too little time on policy process – the 'how' question – and hardly any time at all on implementation – the 'when' question. Three decades of work has produced many policy options, but much of it has been highly technical – the pros and cons of floors and caps, for example – and has not generated a theory of change. It is clear that the choices about how we fund social care are deeply political. There is no technically 'right' or painless answer. This begs the question of whether any more time on evaluating funding options or carrying out yet another review amounts to little more than, at best, gilding the lily, or, at worst, further procrastination. Instead of pursuing the chimera of an optimal policy solution, time and attention should surely now refocus on the politics and process of reform: how to secure sustained political commitment to a clear plan for social care and its delivery and implementation, without the dither and delay that has characterised the story so far.

Fundamentally, this is about politics and the political leadership required to drive reform. Ed Jones is a former special advisor in the Conservative government and was chief of staff to Jeremy Hunt when he was health Secretary. He sums it up:

> There are some issues which will only be resolved if you start with the politics, and the urgent need to sort sustainable social care funding is one of these. We failed in my time in government because we never truly faced up to the stark political choice needed … My own years in government saw an inability or unwillingness to confront those choices. Endless options appraisals and reviews, expert

contributions, industry consultations, and academic exercises were undertaken but we never formed a view, with conviction, about who we were actually willing to upset in order to get this sorted. This is one area where a Prime Minister has to start with a clear political choice and work back from that to the policy mechanism which delivers on it. Simply passing around the same slide decks and evidence reviews which have circulated through Whitehall for more than ten years, expecting a new and easier way through to emerge, is futile. A political call must be taken. One political constituency will have to win out over another. (E. Jones, 2020)

Lesson 7: Take a long-term view

Social care reform is a good illustration of three common features of a public policy change that need a long-term focus as described by the Institute for Government:

1. The costs and benefits of good social care are distributed unevenly over time: preventive services designed to reduce the need for long-term care involve costs that are incurred immediately but the benefits may not be realised for several years down the line. There are better models of long-term care based on housing. They involve weaving together complex capital and revenue funding streams, overcoming planning permission and land issues and thus take time to deliver. Another example is that the cost of services that speed up hospital discharges, or prevent admissions in the first place, are borne by councils, but the benefits fall on the NHS.
2. They are intellectually contested, politically contentious and hard to deliver, as exemplified by the history of social care reform.
3. The causes and effects span government siloes. For social care, this involves the Department of Health and Social Care, the Department for Levelling Up, Housing and Communities (covering local government), Department for Work and Pensions as well as the Treasury and 10 Downing Street and

the Cabinet Office. NHS England also has a big stake in reform. Sustaining policy-making momentum, securing buy-in and reaching agreement is complex and time-consuming. (Ilot et al, 2016)

All of the problems in England's social care system so brutally exposed by COVID-19 have been around for a long time and have deep roots that extend well back into the last century. No amount of piecemeal tinkering will be enough, and it will take many years to design, plan and fully implement the scale of change that is required across so many fronts.

Instead, England's usual approach to the pressures and challenges facing social care has been a succession of short-term, ad hoc initiatives. Even when extra money has been put in, this has not been sustained or consistent. Since the mid-1990s, despite a 5 per cent average real-term increase in spending, annual levels of spending bounced around erratically, from an increase of 10.6 per cent in 2002 to a cut of 0.3 per cent in 2007. Since 2015, it is possible to count at least 11 separate funding announcements, in addition to the annual financial settlement for local government between 2015 and 2020 that covered a variety of funding streams. They include the 'improved' Better Care Fund, an Adult Social Care Support Grant, a Social Care Support Grant (covering children's social care as well), an extra grant to help relieve NHS winter pressures and further additional grants (House of Commons Library, 2020a). While financial support to councils was provided after the outbreak of the coronavirus, most of this was not ring-fenced for social care.

In assessing how well the government had prepared health and social care for COVID-19, the UK's independent financial watchdog for public services, the National Audit Office, has pointed out that additional funding has been used to address immediate needs, not to increase the long-term sustainability of services (NAO, 2020).

Short-termism in funding social care makes it hard if not impossible for councils to make sensible plans that can be realised over several years. The Local Government Association has argued for a three-year funding settlement that would allow councils to develop a medium-term strategy. It points out that, for social care:

> A one-year deal provides absolutely none of the certainty social care desperately needs to be able to plan for beyond the next twelve months. This will make it difficult for the NHS and local government to invest jointly in integrated services aimed at improving health outcomes, reducing health inequalities and increasing the resilience and wellbeing of our communities. (Local Government Association, 2020a)

Short-term, hand-to-mouth, funding makes it much harder to develop innovative solutions to care needs; solutions that, in the long run, will achieve better outcomes for people at a lower cost than traditional services. Instead, it shores up the status quo.

Short-termism is not just a money issue in social care. Much of the debate has been 'in the moment', repeating a familiar cycle of heated speculation by the bodies involved in social care about when the latest Green Paper or other policy document will appear and what will be in it. This is despite evidence of past experience that such a document at best is yet another early staging post on a longer journey. The emergence of the 24-hour news cycle has not helped. Then there is the paradox that politicians need to win elections to get anything done, but getting social care done properly will take much longer than a single parliament. Sociologist Elise Boulding has written about modern societies suffering from what she calls 'temporal exhaustion': 'If one is mentally out of breath all the time from dealing with the present, there is no time left for imagining the future' (Fisher, 2019). Sometimes, lip service is paid to a long-term approach, but it rarely lasts. The policy guidance for the community care reforms in the early 1990s, for example, was entitled 'Community Care – the next decade and beyond', but the decade was barely out before attention had shifted to the next reform initiative.

The limited shelf life of ministers is another hindrance. Since 1997, there have been 15 ministers responsible for social care, with most incumbents lucky to be in post for two years, plus ten Secretaries of State. Many took office with their own ideas, though some appeared to have none. For some, wanting to make their own stamp on the role took precedence over following the paths of their predecessor. It is the policy equivalent of attention deficit disorder.

Japan, currently with the most rapidly ageing population in the world, demonstrates the contrast between short-term and long-term thinking. Whereas in England, preventive services that do not produce immediate results have been among the first targets for financial austerity, Japan has recognised the value of prevention in reducing the need for long-term care by supporting people to live as independently as possible in their own communities. It has gone beyond lip service by actively promoting investment in 'upstream' capacity such as community facilities, volunteering and social support networks. It is, as Natasha Curry explains, 'a good example of how the idea of investment in the long term has become a central priority in a country that really can't afford to be short-termist' (Curry, 2017). Chapter 5 will look in more detail at how other countries have planned and implemented changes over a number of years, making adjustments along the way in response to experience and changing circumstances.

Closer to home, Scotland seems to have avoided England's short-term-initiativitis and has stuck with a broad suite of policies over the last two decades that offer free personal care, closer working with the NHS and self-directed support (an approach to social care that gives people maximum choice and control over the support they receive). Rather than frequent chopping and changing of different policies, a recent review of social care in Scotland seeks to build on what has gone before. The review of social care concluded that Scotland has been committed to these approaches for the last 30 years. 'The problem is not that we do not have good ideas; it is that we have not acted on them at scale and with genuine commitment' (Scottish Government, 2021).

A comparison with the NHS, yet again, is instructive. In the last two decades, it has been able to secure political support for substantial increased investment by setting out a clear prospectus for service reform and improvement over a number of years: the NHS Plan in 2000, the Five Year Forward View in 2014 and the NHS Long Term Plan in 2019.

The advantages of a long-term approach are clear and linked to the case for cross-party cooperation discussed under Lesson 3. The scale of the challenge in developing a very different model of social care, with profound implications for what services and support are offered, who will actually provide the care and how all of this is funded, will take at least a decade to develop and implement effectively. The implementation challenge will be massive and can only be met with flexibility over the economic and political cycle. The financial fortunes of social care have always waxed and waned according to the state of the economy and the public finances. Better times will make it easier to fund social care and other public services more generously. Changes in household income and wealth profiles will also shift over time. A settlement based on assumptions about property-rich baby boomers for example will not work for the millennials who are acquiring property wealth at a much slower rate (Gustafsson, 2019). The mixture of public and private sources will need to be adjusted over time such that individual charges will vary relative to general and local taxation or contribution rates (if we went down the road of social insurance).

Lesson 8: Make a positive case for change

The usual narrative around social care reform has been unremittingly glum. Understanding of social care by the general public is, as we have seen, low (Lesson 4). When it does surface into public consciousness, it is portrayed in ways that are almost always negative, couched in the language of demographic time bombs, a financial burden on the taxpayer, a threat to our personal savings and assets, including even the roof over our head. Whereas we readily recognise that we will need health care at some point in our lives – all of us at the beginning and end of our lives – and value the NHS for offering us peace of mind that it will be there for us, media coverage of social care too often reminds us instead of a life we have no wish to know, riven by crises and close to the tipping point of collapse. The 'serenity' described by Nye Bevan about health care, in Chapter 2, is painfully absent. Media representations of older people conjure up negative images of decline, dependency and frailty, which has prompted the #nomorewrinklyhands campaign on Twitter (Centre for Ageing Better, 2020). People with disabilities are generally viewed through a lens of vulnerability and neediness (Survation, 2021) This contributes to the 'othering' of people with care needs in contrast to the positive and full-throated support for the NHS that we see as 'ours'. For politicians, it is an issue of great risk and toxicity, the 'third rail' of politics tainted by past electoral failure. The positive benefits of good social care for individuals, families, and communities, and its potential to help people live the best lives they can, not to mention the economic value of social care to the national and local economy is drowned out by the chorus of crisis and failure. Coupled with the absence of a clear vision for good care, it brings to mind the words of Neil Crowther, 'shovelling water out of a sinking boat, rather than reaching for the stars' (Crowther, 2021). It is hard to drum up public appetite for change – including tax increases to pay for improvements – when social care is portrayed in such a depressing fashion as an overwhelming problem that is too difficult to address.

Again, we can learn from other countries in developing a positive case for change that stresses not simply the costs of a better system but the benefits to individuals and families, and the value of investment in social care as part of wider economic and social objectives. Japan, for example, made its new social insurance arrangements deliberately generous to attract public support (Curry et al, 2018). Australia's reforms were rooted originally in concerns about national productivity (Productivity Commission, 2011). The UK government's industrial strategy launched in 2017 acknowledged the importance of social care to the economy and offered an opportunity to tell a different story about the value and benefits of good social care and not just its costs (HM Government, 2017). Sadly, it was ditched early in 2021 (*Financial Times*, 2021). The case for a positive narrative for change as part of a new road to reform will be developed further in Chapter 7.

Lesson 9: Encourage realistic expectations

The pressures on the social care system are now so great that impatience for immediate change is understandable. But it is clear that the journey from the current system to the one of our dreams will not happen overnight or in one sweeping big bang. There is no golden bullet in social care reform. Yet the reaction to different proposals over the years offers an apt illustration of Voltaire's aphorism of the perfect being the enemy of the good.

The opposition to the Dilnot reforms is a case in point. Although initially well-received, some seeds of dissent were evident from the outset. The National Pensioners Convention, for example, dismissed the proposals as 'tinkering at the edges' and only a full-blooded National Care Service with free personal care would do (BBC News, 2013). Opposition also came from the political right. In 2012, I found myself on BBC 2's *Newsnight* with John Redwood, who made the familiar argument that the state should not protect the property inheritances of relatively well-off people. Improving the quality of care was a more important priority for public funding (Redwood, 2012). Ironically, the former concern was shared by many on the political left, but for a different reason. Their argument was that protecting people from catastrophic costs did not address the problems of inadequate funding of local authority budgets on which people without savings or assets depended. This view was shared by many charities campaigning for better social care, especially those for working-age people with care needs. They too supported the government's decision to postpone the reforms: 'To introduce a cap without doing anything to address the underfunding of social care would be a recipe for disaster' (Care and Support Alliance, 2015).

The opposition of the Local Government Association was influential, giving the government air cover to walk away from a manifesto commitment. It may be that, as Norman Lamb has suggested, the intricate, technical nature of the proposals did not help and that the social care sector was 'underwhelmed'. There was no 'vision', Lamb recalls:

I thought, 'Right let's get the principle legislated for and then there could be a political debate about where the cap should sit. Lib Dems could argue for a lower cap, the Tories for a higher one – whatever you want.' But the problem was that the sector was underwhelmed; it didn't capture the public imagination. No one had any idea what the Dilnot cap was out there in the public, so it was incredibly easy for the Tories to ditch once they got rid of us. It was hardly noticed when they ditched it. (Elliott, 2021)

In hindsight, a heavy price has been for this lack of unity. Had the Dilnot changes gone ahead in 2016, local authority budgets would be at least £6 billion a year better off; hundreds of thousands of people would have benefited from a more generous means test; many people entering adulthood would now be receiving free care; councils would have a new duty to help people paying for their care by bringing self-funders into the system; and all would have access to better information and advice as a universal right. Arguably most important of all, implementation would have established a landmark principle that, for the first time since the creation of the welfare state in 1948, the state was placing a limit on how much people should have to pay for their social care. Instead, there have been no compensating improvements. The money promised by the Treasury disappeared and the battle for better funding and reform has had to start all over again.

Another example of the perfect being the enemy of the good is the rising, but controversial, groundswell of support for the idea of free personal care (such as for washing and bathing, dressing, continence, mobility and help with eating and drinking, discussed in Chapter 2). Originally put forward by the Royal Commission in 1999, it was rejected by Labour as unaffordable and inequitable. It was not even included as an option in its 2010 consultation. The proposal is now backed by a diverse range of bodies of all political hues and none: the independent Barker Commission, the Institute of Public Policy Research, the House of Lords Economic Affairs Committee, Policy Exchange and two parliamentary select committees. On the face of it, free personal care would level-up entitlement to social care so that all basic care needs are met free at the point of use. This would ease much of the funding boundary between the NHS and social care and the problem of continuing healthcare discussed in Chapter 2. Yet this too is opposed by many in the social care world, fearing that free 'personal' or 'life and limb' care would suck resources away from equally vital provisions like prevention and community supports that enable people to lead a better life. Others argue, like Dilnot, that free personal care would simply shift private costs onto the public purse without doing anything to improve the quality and availability of care for those with limited means. And for others, the fear is that free personal care would shift responsibilities from families, summarised by former Secretary of State for health, Andrew Lansley:

> From a Conservative point of view … the risk is that we end up taxing [a] relatively large amount of people's taxable income in order to provide older people personal care. People keep talking about social care as if it was almost all medical care and a lot of it is personal, for which people would normally expect to pay themselves. It's just that when they become really frail, they can't do it for themselves and their family very often does it. But that's a big problem which we encountered in Scotland, which has made personal care free. If you make all this stuff free families wonder why they do it. So instead of families thinking somebody from your local authority has to come in and do it and that the state ends up paying for it so you get quite a lot of increases. (Elliott, 2021)

Faced with such discordant views within the social care sector itself, no wonder these are echoed within political parties and that the government of the day appears to struggle to make up its mind.

As argued earlier, sustainable reforms that really get to grips with all of the varied problems in social care will take years to achieve and require a comprehensive and wide-ranging package of measures. There is not a binary choice, for example between free personal care and a cap to protect people from catastrophic costs. They are different responses to different problems and not mutually exclusive.

The lessons here for everyone who wants to see better social care, including councils, care providers, charities and groups that speak for and with people with care needs, is to manage expectations of progress realistically and tactically over time. First, expectations of scale, pace and timing of change need to be realistic and the purpose of reform needs to be clear (see Lesson 1). After over two decades of waiting, this should not be difficult. Second, use a tactical approach to secure political and public support for reform. Instead of opposing particular proposals because they will not solve everything for everybody all at once, a more fruitful approach would be to seize opportunities for immediate if limited gains as a stepping-stone to further reform. Had the Dilnot reforms been implemented as planned in 2016, the improvements summarised earlier would have placed social care in a much stronger position to argue the case for further changes. The cause of reform has been poorly served by taking a purist rather than a pragmatic approach to particular policy options.

In summary, there is so much that can be learned from the failure of successive government administrations to sort out social care. However, each one, in the spirit of Peter Cook, has found it easier to repeat history than learn from it. Many of these lessons are reflected in the experiences of other countries, especially those who have been successful in introducing major changes to their care arrangements. This is the subject of the next chapter.

5

Learning from abroad

A case of English exceptionalism?

In trying to understand why England has struggled to sort out the many problems in social care, it is important to look beyond our borders to see how other countries have fared. What light might this throw on our failures? What lessons can we learn from their experience? How do they pay for and provide care and support to their citizens and how, unlike England, have they managed to introduce major reforms to do this? What lessons can be learned from their road to reform?

England is not exceptional in needing to face these issues. Most advanced countries share some common challenges around the availability, quality and sustainability of care services:

- A growing and ageing population. In the European Union (EU), the number of people likely to need care is projected to rise from 30.8 million in 2019 to 38 million by 2050. The number of working-age people for every person aged 65 or over will reduce from 3.3 to only 2 during the next 30 years.
- There are more people with disabilities and long-term health conditions, reflecting better medical care and higher life-expectancy.
- Changing family and population structures and mobility mean that countries can no longer rely, as they have done in the past, on unpaid, informal, family carers. Many countries are experiencing severe shortages in their care workforce.

All face big questions about where the extra care workforce will come from in the future. In the EU area, there are already 6.4 million care jobs, and it is estimated that up to 7 million job openings for health care associate professionals and personal care workers will arise by 2030.

- The costs of care are rising rapidly everywhere and are rising faster than the public funding available to meet them. Most countries are trying to close the gap by focusing resources on people with the highest needs, by increasing user charges and by seeking greater efficiencies in how services are provided, Across the EU, public expenditure on long-term care is projected to increase from 1.7 per cent of GDP in 2019 to 2.5 per cent of GDP in 2050 on average (European Commission, 2021).

Many of these problems have been magnified by the impact of COVID-19. In many countries, death rates in care facilities have been high among both residents and staff. Protecting people with complex health and care needs has been difficult. The pandemic has highlighted long-standing weaknesses in how care services are funded, organised and staffed. England is not on its own in this respect (World Health Organisation, 2020). Nor are the accounts of people using social care described in Chapter 3 are unique to England. The testimony of their counterparts in Australia, for example, described experiences of using care services as 'time consuming, overwhelming, frightening, intimidating' (Royal Commission into Aged Care Quality and Safety (2021).

Neither is England that exceptional in the overall thrust and direction of its policies for social care and health. A common feature of the landscape of care services we share with other developed countries is the dominance of residential and nursing homes. In nearly all OECD (Organisation for Economic Cooperation and Development) countries, most long-term care is provided in these settings and takes up a big chunk of their care budgets. In the Netherlands, Switzerland, Slovenia and France, it accounts for over 70 per cent of long-term care spending. In Belgium and the Scandinavian countries (except Finland), it is lower, with nearer to 40 per cent of their long-term care spending devoted to home care. England is somewhere in the middle (OECD, 2020). Over-reliance on residential and nursing homes is unsustainable because of rising demand and costs of services, and it flies in the face of what most people want. Consequently, the most common and long-standing policy ambition across the developed world is to shift the balance of services away from hospitals and long-term care settings towards care based in people's own homes and communities. Whether it is from the point of view of money, outcomes or public preferences, care at home comes out tops.

Another common goal is integrated care for the increasing numbers of people who have a mixture of physical and mental health conditions, combined with associated care and support needs. Most countries have acknowledged that, for groups such as frail older people and people with multiple chronic conditions, poor coordination of physical health, mental health and social care services is wasteful and leads to worse outcomes (OECD, 2017). Many countries like England have chosen to respond to these changes by trying to personalise services by offering people more choice and control, for example through cash payments like personal budgets or direct payments.

Despite these areas of common ground and shared purpose, there are marked differences between countries in how services and funding are organised to achieve these policies. The choices countries make about these matters are strongly influenced by their history, culture and values. As historians and economists would put it, they are path dependent, that is, they are strongly influenced by key decisions that have gone before. For example, Germany's choice of funding long-term care in 1995 was through a new social insurance scheme. This reflected its historical use of social insurance for old-age pensions, originally introduced by Bismarck in the 1880s, and later for health care (Cylus et al, 2018). Across the developed world, there is much variation between countries and particular quirks in their approaches to long-term care. A key difference between countries is the extent to which the risk, and therefore the costs, of individuals needing a lot of care, are shared or 'pooled' across the whole population. This is what Winston Churchill meant in 1911 when he described compulsory insurance against unemployment as bringing the 'magic of averages to the rescue of millions' (a term recently used by Prime Minister Johnson in the context of social care) (Golding, 2020). Risk-pooling is an important principle of social care reform, because, as discussed in Chapter 4, none of us know the likelihood of needing social care, how much of it we will need and how much it will cost (for a concise explanation of risk-pooling see Nuffield Trust, 2019).

Despite the many differences between countries in their policies on long-term care, it is nevertheless possible to group them into three very broad models:

- In Nordic countries, long-term care is part of a state-run welfare system in which services are universally available, funded largely through general taxation and highly regulated. The level of provision available is relatively generous. Co-payments (the charges paid by individual users) are relatively low – everyone contributes to the collective costs of care, irrespective of whether they will need it, through general taxation. This means that, in these countries, risk-pooling across the whole population is very high, with public support for relatively high levels of personal taxation in return for high levels of public services, including long-term care. It is usually the case that most of the general taxation is raised locally, with central government grants used to iron out differences between places in how much revenue can be raised.

- Northern and central European countries and some Far East countries also offer a relatively universal level of care provision, and a very high level of risk-pooling, but this is achieved through compulsory social insurance rather than general taxation. Such schemes give individuals a right or an 'entitlement' to a pre-defined level of support (in services or cash). This depends on the person's needs, in return for defined contributions or premiums. These are usually deducted at source from wages and salaries. It is common for people without children to pay a slightly higher rate on the assumption that children would provide some degree of informal care for their parents. Employers are also required to contribute to the fund. Examples of countries with well-established formal social insurance schemes are Germany, France, Japan and South Korea. Even free-market Singapore auto-enrols workers into age-care insurance, although they can opt out later.

- Southern and eastern European and Latin American countries rely heavily on informal and unpaid family care, with the state offering a very basic safety net through taxation or social insurance. In these countries, risk-pooling is very low, with much of the cost falling on the shoulders of individuals and families.

This is a broad categorisation. Most countries use a mixture of funding sources; a mixture that is in a state of flux because of rising demand and higher costs. Japan, acclaimed for its reforms of care funding, has come to rely more on general taxation, which now amounts to almost half of its spending on long-term care. Similarly, Korea's social insurance scheme meets only 60 to 65 per cent of its long-term care spending; the remainder coming from government subsidy and co-payments. Some eastern European countries seem to be developing into hybrid welfare states, with strong reliance on family support and a tradition of residential care.

In many European countries, responsibilities for long-term care are shared between national, regional and local government bodies. In those with compulsory social insurance schemes, entitlements to care, funding and assessment of individual needs are more likely to be determined centrally, though assessments are often delegated to local municipalities.

A shift towards the outsourcing of care to private companies is a discernible trend, even in high-spending countries with a strong tradition of universal public provision. Since the 1990s, the share of services provided by private (for-profit) organisations has increased from virtually zero to 18 to 19 per cent in Finland and Sweden and to around 4 to 6 per cent in Denmark and Norway. In none of these countries has the not-for-profit sector grown. Sweden has moved fastest towards outsourcing, but most services are still publicly provided. Private companies provide just 19 per cent of all home care services and 20 per cent of long-term residential care (Szebehely and Meagher, 2018).

England (and to a certain extent Wales, Scotland and Northern Ireland) do not fit particularly well into any of these three broad groupings. Although it shares with most countries the high-level goals of promoting independence and offering more care to people in their own homes instead of long-term care facilities, beyond the rhetoric, England is exceptional for all the wrong reasons. As described in Chapter 3, the state offers no more than a basic safety net for the most essential needs. It was never really part of the universal welfare state established in the 1940s, and a decade of austerity from 2010 has further eroded the level of provision. There is heavy reliance on general taxation to pay for care, but access to publicly funded care is also tightly restricted to the poorest through a draconian means test. The degree of social protection afforded to people by the state is very limited indeed. People with many care needs are exposed to 'catastrophic' costs and these significantly reduce the incomes of working-age disabled people, who lose some of their disability benefits to pay for care. As in many southern European countries, and parts of the developing world, much of the responsibility of care sits with families. So, England is neither one thing nor another. The extent to which the costs of care are pooled across the whole population is minimal compared with many similar countries. In this respect, England has more in common with the USA in its long-term care arrangements. We are also an outlier in having over 90 per cent of care services provided by private and voluntary organisations.

The most glaring case of English exceptionalism is that, while many countries have faced up to challenges of changing needs and rising costs by making major changes to their care systems, governments here have dithered and delayed. In 1968, the Netherlands introduced social insurance for long-term care and went on to make further reforms in 2015. In 1992, Sweden devolved responsibilities for long-term care to local authorities, with financial incentives to reduce the use of institutional care (the Ädel reforms). In 1995, Germany introduced compulsory social insurance to cover long-term care needs, as did Japan five years later for people over 40. In both countries, these arrangements built on their long tradition of compulsory health insurance. France followed in 2002 with its own version, the Allocation Personnalisée Autonomie (APA). Korea was next in 2008, adding long-term care to its existing national health insurance programme. Spain transformed its long-term care system with the introduction of its System for Promotion of Personal Autonomy and Assistance for Persons in Situation of Dependency (SAAD). In 2009, Ireland reformed means-testing with the Nursing Home Support Scheme, which limited how much people had to pay towards nursing home costs. In 2013, Australia legislated to give older people more control over their care plans, better access to care services and more generous means-testing, including a cap on care costs. At the same time, it introduced a national disability insurance scheme to provide a range of support to people with disabilities of all ages, including children.

To understand the differences and similarities between countries in respect of long-term care, it is helpful to look in more detail at what they do.

Continental Europe

In France, Germany and the Netherlands, care needs are seen as a universal risk, best handled by pooling across the whole population. Germany and the Netherlands do this through a mandatory social insurance scheme, while France has opted for one main care benefit funded through general taxation, the APA. This is universal, but not necessarily generous. Social insurance schemes in France and Germany are explicitly designed to cover only a part of the costs of the care, with remaining costs met by the individual through co-payments, private insurance or funding from the local municipality.

The Netherlands established a compulsory universal social insurance scheme for social care needs in 1968, called AWBZ. This is administered by private insurance companies. It is paid for via an income-related premium deducted from the wages of all citizens aged 16 and over, plus an employer contribution through payroll taxes. In response to escalating costs, the Dutch long-term care system underwent significant reform in 2015, and the AWBZ was split into parts. Residential care is now available under a new Long-term Care Act; replacing AWBZ as the primary scheme for long-term care and absorbed most of its funding. Home nursing care is now part of the basic Health

Insurance Act and the responsibility of health insurers, while municipalities have taken on responsibility for most forms of non-residential care through the Social Support Act. The level of provision is very generous: until recently, help with housework, for example, was included in care packages. The use of residential and nursing care is high. In 2019, the Netherlands spent 3.7 per cent of its GDP on long-term care, the highest of any OECD country (OECD, 2021).

Germany's universal social insurance scheme, introduced in 1995, covers older people and disabled people of working age. Based on the country's long-standing health insurance scheme, members are enrolled automatically into it. Contributions are raised through a mandatory income tax and shared between employee and employer. In 2020, the contribution rate was 3.05 per cent of gross income, shared equally between employers and employees. The scheme is intended to cover basic needs only, with a strong expectation that individuals and families should contribute significantly to both the cost of care and its provision. People without children, who are less likely to receive informal support, are required to pay an extra 0.25 per cent (soon to be increased to 0.35 per cent), and benefits that are taken in cash rather than services are reduced. Everyone can opt for private insurance instead, but these products are highly regulated (premiums cannot be higher than the public scheme). The cost of accommodation is not included, and services are not funded until six months after needs have been assessed. For those unable to contribute their share of the costs, there is a means-tested safety net operated by the federal states. By the end of 2018, around 89 per cent of the population was insured under the statutory insurance scheme, while around 11 per cent held a private long-term care insurance policy.

So, although Germany's scheme is universal, it relies heavily on co-payment. This may explain why its public spending on long-term care is relatively low compared with many of its neighbours. At just 1.5 per cent of GDP in 2019, it is the same as the UK. Germany's approach offers everybody something, but is not necessarily generous or without cost to the individual, especially for residential care. Similar to most countries with statutory social insurance schemes, Germany has had to hike contribution rates at least nine times since 1995 to address rises in costs and the numbers of people entitled to care. It now plans, for the first time, to inject some general tax funding to help with the costs, so it will cease to be a 'pure' social insurance scheme.

Germany's reforms have also included measures to ensure a sustainable provider market by combining nationally set benefits and state-level legal frameworks with local price negotiations (European Commission, 2021a). More recently, it has decided to introduce a monthly cap to help protect people from rising costs (Schlepper, 2021).

France stands out from other countries in that support is delivered through several different channels. Its central benefit is the APA, which is for anyone aged 60 or over who needs help with activities of daily living, either in their own homes or care homes. The amount of benefit is adjusted according to the individual's level of need and income level. The assessment is based on seven levels of dependency and is carried out by a multidisciplinary team employed by *départements* (a regional tier of administration) who use the scheme's benefit to fund a care plan.

Although the APA is a universal benefit, it covers only a proportion of the costs of care. In addition, France has several smaller types of health insurance and pension schemes that can help with social care costs. There are various tax reliefs related to disability and the purchase of residential and home care, and some people may get long-term care through their health insurance, although it is not clear how widely this is available. In addition, 15 per cent of over-40s have private long-term care insurance, usually because it has been bundled in with their supplementary (*mutuelle*) health insurance. However, these policies do not in general cover the full cost of care and instead make only small payments when people become disabled (OECD, 2011). As a result, private insurance plays only a very small role in protecting people from the cost of care.

The complexity of the French system makes it difficult for care users and policy-makers alike to assess the adequacy of the social protection it provides, although there seems be a consensus that APA payments are too low. It is also notable that, despite having more universal elements in its long-term care system,

France's spending as a percentage of GDP, at 1.9 per cent, is mid-table. Both the funding and governance is challenging to understand, with responsibilities split between health and long-term care but also between the state (central government, regions, *départements* and municipalities). The absence in France of a means-tested safety net for care at home appears to create a perverse incentive for people to enter residential care earlier than they would otherwise need to. It is of note that older people in France have relatively high incomes compared with many other countries, so, someone with median pension income could spend nearly half of their income on care before they reached the poverty threshold. France has continued to make changes and adjustments: since 2017, for example, tax credits are available to people employing their own carers. Following the Libault Report in 2019, France is planning a further wave of reform to rationalise funding, expand and improve home care and residential facilities, and provide more support to informal carers (European Commission, 2021a).

Scandinavia

Sweden typifies the Scandinavian approach in relying primarily on taxation, especially local taxation, to fund both health and social care, and the level of co-payment through user charges is very modest. About 90 per cent of care costs are met by local taxation levied by the municipalities: national taxation covers 5 per cent, and the remainder comes from user contributions. The latter is determined on the basis of income alone: the value of property and other assets are not taken into account. There is a ceiling on fees. In 2020, the maximum monthly charge for home care was €195 and for residential care €200. Heavy reliance on taxation and generous levels of provision explain why Sweden spent 3.2 per cent of its GDP on long-term care in 2019. This is on a par with its Nordic neighbours.

Budget pressures have been managed by reducing the use of residential care. The proportion of older people living in residential care has fallen from 22 per cent in 1993 to around 12 per cent in 2017. Sweden seems to have maintained a very high and generous level of home care services, including help with housework and shopping, as does the Netherlands. These are services that most English local authorities ceased to provide long ago. Sweden experiences familiar workforce pressures, but its recruitment and retention rates are among the highest in the OECD. Care workers' pay is around 70 per cent of average salary levels (which in Sweden are high) (European Commission (2021a). It is one of the few countries that has successfully expanded its care workforce in recent years (OECD, 2021a).

A particular feature of the Scandinavian approach is that responsibility for long-term care is highly decentralised. Local authorities are responsible not only for assessing each person's needs and arranging care but raising the money locally as well. There are no nationally imposed eligibility criteria. To UK localists, this may sound like paradise, but there are downsides. The Swedish equivalent of attendance allowance and carers' allowance – that in England offer important financial support for people with care needs – are subject to a local needs assessment, and municipalities can decide not to offer these benefits at all.

Although Sweden's overall approach to managing the coronavirus has attracted great interest, its long-term care facilities seem to have been as badly hit as many other countries. The interim conclusions of a government-established commission of inquiry makes for familiar reading, attributing the impact on care services to fragmented responsibilities between local, regional and national authorities, poor access to personal protective equipment and insufficient staff, especially nursing staff (Statens Offentliga Utredningar, 2021). So, despite its generosity and universalism, Sweden should not necessarily be regarded uncritically as the El Dorado of international care systems.

Arguably the most interesting aspect of Sweden's care system is its claim that the care needs of its older people have reduced since the 1980s because of better health (Swedish Government, 2021). It gives high priority to preventive health care and supporting activities that help people remain independent and socially engaged, instead of focusing narrowly on personal care. Life expectancy in Sweden is among the highest in the world: 80.6 years for men and 84.3 years for women.

Japan

Japan is often cited as a country that has successfully implemented major reforms in how it funds and delivers long-term care, this while facing a perfect storm of one the oldest populations in the world, a declining birth rate, sluggish economic growth and a high national debt. It had significant problems with inadequate and unaffordable long-term care and heavy reliance on informal family carers. Care costs were rising rapidly. Earlier reforms – the ten-year Gold Plan in 1989 – had not worked that well (Ikegami, 2007).

The Long-Term Care Insurance (LTCI) scheme was introduced in 2000. It offers universal, comprehensive care to people over the age of 65 and those with a disability aged between 40 and 65, regardless of wealth or income. Instead of focusing solely on people with very high personal care needs, it aims to prevent care and health needs by funding services that promote independence and wellbeing, such as exercise classes and community centres. Around 50 per cent of its funding comes from a mixture of national and local taxation. The other half comes from insurance premiums. For people over 65 (the 'primary insured'), these are deducted from pension payments by municipalities; for 40–65-year-olds, they are collected through social insurance arrangements that were already in place, before these reforms, for health care. Employers contribute to the premiums. For the average citizen, contributions amounted to 1.5 per cent of their monthly income. Japan has also modified the structure of insurance premiums so they are fairer. There is a monthly cap on individual contributions to care home costs.

Japan's is a mixed funding model, with the money channelled to municipalities that assess each person's needs against seven levels of eligibility on a nationally determined scale. This in turn determines a notional budget for that person's needs, which is used by a care manager to agree with them a package of care to meet their needs. The care manager is usually employed by a care provider, though the individual is able to request a different person of their own choosing. There is no financial means-testing or financial assessment as such, but a means-tested accommodation charge was introduced in 2005.

In the early years of the new scheme, demand and costs rose sharply from 3.6 yen in 2000 to 10.7 trillion yen in 2017. This was largely because more people were eligible for help than had been expected, especially those with relatively low levels of need. The balance between needs and costs has been regulated strategically through a review of needs and resources every three years. This has led to people with low needs being limited to preventive support only. User contributions have been increased several times, especially for those with higher incomes: those with an income of 3.4 million yen (around £22,500) or more were paying a 30 per cent co-payment from 2018. And there have been regular increases in insurance premiums, although average contributions still remain below 2 per cent of average income.

Natasha Curry and colleagues at the Nuffield Trust have spent time in Japan looking at how their approach has worked and what lessons could be learned for England. They highlight the importance of requiring contributions from the age of 40, when many people become aware of the importance of the benefits of good care for their ageing parents. They further highlight the establishment of generous national entitlements and eligibility levels, which have made it possible to secure public support for the new system, and, crucially, willingness to pay for it (Curry et al, 2018). There is an interesting observation by Camilla Cavendish, former head of the 10 Downing Street policy unit, in her book *Extra Time*:

> Talking to younger Japanese, I found that many seem to have more faith in long-term care insurance than in their state pensions. One expert told me that his own son no longer pays into his pension. Governments have tinkered too much, he said. They think the pension will have vanished by the time they grow old, but the care scheme seems more stable – and fair. (Cavendish, 2019)

The most interesting aspect of care reform in Japan is the breadth of its approach, looking beyond the narrow question of how to pay for long-term care services. As in Sweden, Japan has encouraged investment in community facilities that prevent ill-health and promote activity and social engagement. The government has addressed a long-term strategy for 'community-based integrated care systems' based not only on formal services provided by health and care organisations but also on mutual support from local communities (England's fledgling Integrated Care Systems should take note). Municipalities are given 3 per cent of the total long-term care budget, a ring-fenced amount to pay for local prevention and support. This also includes making provision for those who are not eligible for care under the long-term care insurance scheme (Hayashi, 2011). The key point here is that, in Japan, prevention is seen as a major plank in its long-term strategy to make sure that the long-term care system is sustainable – by preventing and reducing the need for formal health and care services in the first place. In contrast, in England, preventive services and support for community facilities have usually been the first to be sacrificed to make savings.

Japan's reform programme also looked at the supply side of care and how providers can be encouraged to offer quality and choice in ways that are financially sustainable. It should be noted here that the provider market in Japan comprises large numbers of small and local organisations. Payments to providers are set according to a national fee schedule with seven unit-price levels that include an adjustment for local costs. This has enabled the government to shape the overall balance of provision and exercise some control over costs. In the early days of the new scheme, fee rates for hospitals, for example, were lowered and those for community providers were raised to encourage a shift in care away from institutional settings. A very centralised approach has not been without its problems: some municipalities argued for higher fee levels to make it easier for providers to meet needs in their area, and there are concerns that a tight control on fees may not cover provider costs and so cause them to leave the market (as has been the case in England).

Lower fees have also led to lower care staff wage levels compared with the rest of the economy, exacerbating growing staff shortages in care services. Japan does not have the impact of Brexit hanging over its care workforce, but neither does it have a strong tradition of immigration to meet its staffing gaps (Curry et al, 2018).

Australia

Australia is a particularly interesting example because the reforms it introduced from 2012 – the Aged Care (Living Longer Living Better) Act – were prompted by similar weaknesses that afflict England's care system. These included a fragmented system, with complex means-testing rules that made it hard for people to understand and navigate. However, the level of service appeared to be more generous than England (Australian Government, 2012; Forder and Fernandez, 2011b). The government considered but rejected compulsory social insurance and private insurance. Instead, Australia has opted to continue with a mixture of general taxation and a more generous blend of means-tested fees and charges for specific services. Significantly, this included a cap on care costs not dissimilar to that proposed by the Dilnot Commission (discussed in Chapter 4). In Australia, the maximum amount anyone has to contribute towards their residential care costs is $28,339 annually, with a lifetime cap of $68,102 (as of July 2021) – equivalent to around £15,000 and £36,000 (Australian Government, 2021). These are much lower – and more generous – limits than the figures touted in England. Older people who use aged care services pay for about a quarter of the total cost of those services. The 2012 reforms also introduced a new national gateway into the system to get information and access to services, the 'My Aged Care' platform.

Australia has shifted towards a much more centralised model. The government in Canberra is directly responsible for most aspects of policy, planning and funding, including even controlling the number of residential places and home-care packages. There is a fixed ratio per 100,000 population for both services, as well as for paying providers. The role played by states and territories is now much more limited compared with local authorities in England. People's needs are assessed by around 80 Aged Care Assessment Teams (ACAT) operating across Australia, based either in hospitals or in the local community (Australian Institute of Health and Welfare, 2018).

Australia is also noteworthy because it introduced quite separate reforms for people with disabilities who have long-term support needs, including children. Introduced in 2013, this is the National Disability Insurance Scheme (NDIS). To people with a significant and permanent disability, it offers services and forms of support they need to live and enjoy their lives. An explicit aim of the NDIS is to give all Australians peace of mind that if their child or relative is born with or acquires a significant disability, they will get the support they need. It does this by pooling risks across the population and taking the risk of disability support costs away from individuals and families. Funding is shared across the national, state and territory governments, largely through general taxation. This is based on actuarial estimates of long-term spending. Operated by an independent government agency, the National Disability Insurance Agency (NDIA), the scheme works with local partners, usually through an area coordinator, to agree with each participant an individual plan that sets out their goals and funding. Goals might include volunteering, getting and keeping a job, making friends or participating in a local community activity. The scope of the scheme is unusual in going beyond traditional personal care to involve help with activities of daily living, insisting that 'NDIS is not a welfare system' (National Disability Insurance Agency, 2021). Compared with aged care, NDIS offers more comprehensive support, with greater access to specialised care, aids, equipment and therapy. The average amount of available funding is often greater.

Evaluations of both sets of reforms have demonstrated clear improvements. Coverage of services has become more generous. Around a third of the older population use publicly funded care, a number that has been rising steadily over the last decade. For most people this takes the form of low-level support, including home maintenance and cleaning, meals and transport services. The numbers of people getting support through the NDIS has also soared. These undoubted improvements have come at a price, however. For people of all ages, the growth in numbers and costs has caused worries about the financial sustainability of both the NDIS and aged care programmes. There have been continuing concerns about variations in access to support, waiting times and the quality of care. The entitlements that people with disabilities have under the NDIS scheme appear to be more generous than those for older people under the aged care programme (a cautionary note about having separate systems for working-age disabled people and older people). The payment system for residential care for older people remains very complicated, especially for accommodation costs (Davy, 2019).

The phased implementation of NDIS across Australia has been complex and challenging in terms of the sheer number of assessments, described as 'a tsunami of new participants', and concerns about their quality and that of the resulting support plans (Productivity Commission, 2017). Developing the capacity of services and the workforce to meet these needs has also been problematic. But there remains strong support for what the scheme is trying to achieve and its ambition to offer disabled people a better life. As one disability advocate put it:

> I have seen the life changes in people with disability who now have NDIS funding. They are now accessing community, having a good life and have hope for their futures. The burdens are off the family, some aged carers, and there is job creation. Broken wheelchairs are now being replaced and people who never had wheelchairs, now have and can access the community. I now see happy people. (Productivity Commission, 2017)

An independent review in 2018 recommended that the cap on care costs for older people should be abolished, but this has yet to be accepted. In the following year, the government made a commitment that no one under the age of 65 should enter residential aged care from 2022, and that no one under the age of 65 should live in residential aged care from 2025. A wider assessment by the Royal Commission on Aged Care Quality and Safety in 2020 recommended further changes to both schemes, with the government accepting most, but by no means all, of the its recommendations (Australian Government, 2021a). The government has yet to make up its mind on whether personal care, social support (including transport), home modifications and assistive technologies should be free at the point of use and in effect replace the current annual and lifetime cap on care costs. But the commission did accept that people should still be expected to contribute to their accommodation and living costs.

The royal commission has led to a major new reform programme, the Aged Care Act 2021, with a funding package of $18 billion (Australian Government, 2021a). This will enshrine in law a set of universal principles, including the rights to high-quality, safe and timely support and care, and protection from unsafe and harmful 'care'. In addition, it will establish an independent pricing authority to set fees for care services, and a new aged care programme that brings together existing services that hitherto had operated separately (the Commonwealth Home Support Programme, Home Care Packages Program and Residential Aged Care Program and including respite care and short-term restorative care.)

Setting aside the detailed impact of these measures, the key point for this discussion is that, like many other countries, Australia's reforms have not solved every problem all at once. That many more people are getting support has created fresh challenges around funding and financial sustainability. Further changes have been necessary in the light of experience and evidence. Australia's used of periodic reviews and independent commissions to inform these is of note.

Spending compared: apples and pears?

Trying to make sense of how England's approach to social care compares with other countries is fraught with problems, especially when it comes to money. Chapter 3 described how in England social care means different things to different people and how the terminology has changed so much over the years. The term social care is rarely used outside the UK, instead 'long-term care' (LTC) is the preferred nomenclature.

These difficulties are multiplied when we look at how other countries interpret these matters. It does not help that the foremost consideration seems to be to collect and classify data that enables health care expenditure for each country to be compared consistently. This system of 'health accounts' was introduced in 2011 and is followed by the EU, the OECD and the WHO. It talks about 'long-term care' which is defined as:

The range of services required by persons with a reduced degree of functional capacity, physical or cognitive, and who are consequently dependent for an s extended period of time on help with basic activities of daily living (ADL) such as bathing, dressing, eating, getting in and out of bed or chair, moving around and using the bathroom. (OECD, 2017a)

This is more or the less the same as the very functional definition of social care as personal care: being 'fed, cleaned and watered' – the basic activities of daily living including help with washing, dressing and so on described in Chapter 3. These come under the OECD category of 'long-term care (health)'. When this definition was first applied to the UK from 2014, an immediate consequence was that a fair chunk of NHS spending, such as on district nursing, nursing homes and palliative care, was reclassified as long-term care spending. This change appeared to add 1.5 per cent to the NHS's share of GDP, but this was an accounting change only – the actual money spent was unchanged (Appleby, 2016).

The OECD framework also includes another category called 'long-term care (social)', covering a wider range of support, beyond personal care, that helps people to live independently, including help with daily living such shopping, laundry, cooking, housework and social activities. Sometimes they are referred to as 'instrumental activities of daily living' or IADLs. Unfortunately, some countries do not report these figures, and others include them in the long-term care (health) category (Mueller et al, 2020).

Where England (and to a large extent other UK jurisdictions) does stand apart from many other countries is that, since the 2014 Care Act, it has adopted a much broader definition of social care. The Act defines social care in terms of the outcomes needed to achieve individual wellbeing rather than particular kinds of need or services. In theory at least, the assessments of people's care needs should be 'strengths-based', that is, based on the individual's aspirations. In contrast, entitlements under social insurance schemes are determined more through deficits – the help someone needs with ADLs and IADLs.

The important point here is that these definitions do not always reflect how things are done in England, or in other countries, where the boundary between health and care services are fuzzy and are the responsibility of different organisations at different levels of national, regional and local government.

Looking at how much countries spend on long-term care is inevitably hedged with caution and caveats. On the face of it, the UK (separate data is not submitted for England or the devolved administrations) does not look too bad, with public spending on long-term care (both health and social as defined by the OECD) about 1.5 per cent of its GDP in 2019 (Figure 5.1). This places us just above the average across all of these countries, and on a par with wealthy countries like Canada and Germany. But, as noted, this is based on a definition of long-term care that includes a big chunk of NHS spending, so it makes England look more munificent than it is. Setting aside the OECD definitions, UK public spending on adult social care, based on what councils spend, is about 1.1 per cent of GDP. It also appears that some countries – notably Australia and the United States – under-report their spending on all kinds of long-term care by a very big margin and the reporting of the social category of long-term care spending is very patchy. None of these figures include private spending on care, through co-payments or user charges, which can make a significant difference to overall spending by each country. It is not surprising that poorer countries spend a lot less, but, even among richer countries, there are big differences, as Figure 5.1 shows.

And the answer is?

There is no evidence that any one country has comprehensively addressed and resolved every single one of the challenges they face in delivering and funding long-term care. None can offer a neat template of a perfect social care system. Recruiting and retaining enough care workers with the right skills and aptitude seems to be a continuing problem for most if not all countries. Nor is it possible to identify an ideal funding system that ticks every box (Robertson et al, 2014). In all countries, the choice of funding methods is intrinsically political and is shaped by

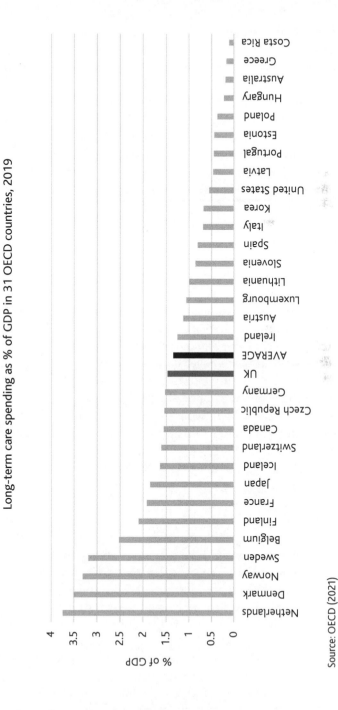

Figure 5.1: What countries spend on long-term care

Long-term care spending as % of GDP in 31 OECD countries, 2019

Source: OECD (2021)

each country's traditions and previous choices: they are path dependent. COVID-19 has prompted fresh thinking in many countries, such as Germany, France, Luxembourg, Netherlands, Slovakia and Slovenia, about what further changes are needed, but in Belgium and Finland, planned changes have been put on hold (European Social Network, 2021). There is some evidence that countries with less developed long-term care systems, especially in Europe, have expanded their coverage and become more generous. In contrast, countries with universal long-term care models have moved in the opposite direction, towards what has been described as 'restricted universalism' (Ranci and Pavolini, 2015). This raises the question of whether countries in the long term are converging towards a mixture of funding approaches (Gori et al, 2016).

As England continues to be struggle with thorny choices about the future of social care, the experience of many other countries offers some very clear learning points. This is especially so with regard to how they have secured public and political support, the Achilles heel of English endeavours. Perhaps the most obvious is the way in which other countries have begun their road to reform from a positive starting point, rooted in wider positive social and economic policy objectives. In Australia, the impetus for reform came from two inquires carried out by the country's Productivity Commission, an independent advisory body that looks at a wide range of policy issues to do with economic performance and community wellbeing. The scope and ambition of its final report on aged care is striking:

> The overriding objective of public policy is to improve the wellbeing of the community as a whole. In the context of aged care policy, the focus for older people should be on their physical and emotional needs, connectedness to others, ability to exert influence over their environment, and their safety – within their expressed life choices. At a broader level, the wellbeing of family members, friends and neighbours who provide care to older people, and people who provide formal care also need to be considered. (Productivity Commission, 2011a)

Australia's NDIS was also justified in terms of the economic benefits to individuals and society, such as participation in the labour market, the wellbeing of disabled people and their carers, efficiency gains and savings by other public services. The commission described the economic benefits of the new scheme as 'profound' and easily exceeding its costs (Productivity Commission, 2011).

Sweden argues that, because of its high spending on social protection and public health, the population is healthier and has lower long-term care needs. Japan used its economic problems as a reason to promote care reform, not an excuse to postpone or delay it. Much of the impetus behind Germany's reforms was propelled by the social and economic challenges of reunification. They were intended to promote prevention, independence and social inclusion, not just meet a narrow range of care needs (Curry et al, 2019).

The experience of these countries underlines the importance of the lesson in the previous chapter about asking the right question or questions about the purpose of reform and what it is meant to achieve. In other words, if social care reform is the answer, what is the question? In contrast, in England, the question has been framed in a very singular way, expressed in the language of crisis, costs and dependency. The 'problem' of social care has usually focused almost exclusively on how to protect the value of people's houses from care charges. The underpinning narrative frames care as a threat to personal wealth or inheritances, and an assumption that choices about care funding will always be toxic and unpopular. As noted in the previous chapter, the purpose and benefits of good social care have become disconnected and sidelined by a sole fixation on the hard choices about how and by whom social care is paid for. That is not to say that funding and costs have been unimportant in other countries, but they have been viewed in the context of wider objectives where there has been as much attention to the benefits of good social care. That in turn has helped to build public and political support for reforms instead of frightening voters with talk of death and dementia taxes.

While England has fretted about money and inheritances, Table 5.1 shows how, over just three years, many European

Table 5.1: Long-term care reforms in European countries, 2017–2020

Member state	Long-term care cash benefits for the dependent person			Homecare services			Residential (or semi-residential) services			Informal carers				Workforce		
	LTC cash benefits for the dependent person	Access	Affordability	Quality	Financing	Access	Affordability	Quality	Financing	Cash benefits	Leave	Employment conditions	Other support	Recruitment	Salary and working conditions	Training and up-skilling
Belgium	×	×		×	×	×		×	×	×	×		×			×
Bulgaria	×	×	×		×	×		×								×
Czech Republic	×									×	×	×			×	
Denmark				×				×						×		
Germany	×	×	×	×	×	×	×	×	×	×			×	×	×	×
Estonia		×		×	×	×		×	×		×		×		×	×
Ireland		×				×				×			×			
Greece		×														
Spain											×		×			
France								×		×			×			
Croatia											×			×	×	
Italy	No reforms during the period under examination															
Cyprus		×	×		×	×										
Latvia		×		×				×					×			
Lithuania				×												
Luxembourg			×	×	×		×	×	×				×		×	

Table 5.1: Long-term care reforms in European countries, 2017–2020 (continued)

Member state	Long-term care cash benefits for the dependent person			Homecare services			Residential (or semi-residential) services			Informal carers				Workforce		
	LTC cash benefits for the dependent person	Access	Affordability	Quality	Financing	Access	Affordability	Quality	Financing	Cash benefits	Leave	Employment conditions	Other support	Recruitment	Salary and working conditions	Training and up-skilling
Hungary	X	X				X				X						
Malta		X	X	X		X		X					X	X		X
The Netherlands				X	X		X	X	X				X		X	X
Austria	X					X	X		X		X					
Poland	X	X	X		X				X	X						
Portugal				X						X	X		X			
Romania		X			X			X				X	X			
Slovenia	No reforms during the period under examination															
Slovakia				X	X	X	X	X	X	X	X					
Finland		X	X	X	X	X	X	X					X	X		
Sweden		X			X	X			X					X		X

Source: European Commission (2021)

countries have worked to improve care services across several fronts – home care, residential care, informal carers and workforce. It is not just about fixing the money.

Another factor behind the progress of other countries is that, for them, health care and social care are mostly funded in a broadly similar way. This made it much easier for them to introduce social insurance because this was how they already funded health care, with which the public were familiar; it did not involve a radical administrative and policy shift. In England, however, there is a stark contrast between very comprehensive and universal funding of health care and extensive rationing and means-testing of social care. That we have chosen to fund social care in a completely different and less generous way than health care has unnecessarily manufactured problems at the boundary of the two services. The huge difference in funding and individual entitlements has created all sorts of problems (discussed in Chapter 3), such as the Berlin Wall of continuing healthcare. This makes it harder for people to leave hospital with the right support and gets in the way of offering well-coordinated services to people who have a mixture of health and care needs. Although many countries find it difficult to offer integrated care, this is usually because of fragmented organizational and professional responsibilities rather than funding.

Just how important is the amount of money a country spends on long-term care? It is clear from Figure 5.1 that most countries similar to England spend a lot more than we do. Even allowing for the risk of comparing apples and pears, England does appear to be at the wrong end of the OECD league table. There is deep concern about the impact of austerity and funding cuts on social care in England. A frequent refrain in the English debate is that 'it's not all about the money.' This is indeed correct. Ironically, there is a risk that funding reform on its own would *worsen* the problems in social care by perpetuating poor-quality services that no longer meet people's changing needs and aspirations. Throwing more money at a complex system that is hard to understand and use, offers limited choices, variable quality and too often fails to meet people's wish to live in their own home is hardly likely to make things better. But, while money is not everything, as Alex Fox has pointed out, better social care is simply not possible without more of it (Fox, 2018).

An even more interesting question than how much countries spend on long-term care is how well they spend it. Here it is clear that some countries are smart spenders. Older people in Sweden, Japan and Australia with relatively low levels of need are much more likely to draw on preventive and support resources in their own communities, whereas in England spending is focused heavily on those with the highest needs. Big spending is not necessarily smart spending. The Netherlands has sustained very high numbers of nursing home places at the expense of supporting people to live at home, although this is now changing.

Another clear message from other countries is that the introduction of more generous and comprehensive access to public funding almost always leads to rising costs as more people are drawn into the system. This is on top of existing cost pressures, such as demography and higher wages. This was the case after the introduction of free personal care in Scotland and compulsory social insurance in Germany and Japan. In the latter case, entitlements to the scheme were deliberately designed to be generous to garner public support for the changes, a strategy that appears to have worked. The price of success has been a bigger bill, and the reaction to this is interesting: in most countries the debate has not been about undoing the reforms or dramatically scaling back entitlements but how to preserve the benefits while finding different ways of making the funding more sustainable. There is no sign, for example, of Scotland reversing its policy on free personal care. On the contrary, in 2019, it was extended to people aged under 65 through 'Frank's Law', after the former Dundee United footballer Frank Kopel, who was diagnosed with dementia at the age of 59 and died six years later in 2014. Germany or Japan have no intention of abandoning their long-term care insurance schemes, each over 20 years old, or Australia unpicking its NDIS or aged care reforms. Instead, the focus of policy thinking and debate in these countries is about adjustment, recalibration and building on the reforms already in place. This suggests that, although landmark legislation is necessary, it will not be sufficient to achieve real change – this involves a continuous cycle of implementation, review and adjustment or further reform. In comparison, England has barely reached first base.

So, there is much we can learn from the processes that other countries have used to reform their care systems. A final observation is that almost all have taken a long-term view and it has often taken years, in some cases over a decade, to design and plan the reforms and secure the public and political support to implement them. In these countries, reform has been viewed as a continuing process rather than a one-off change. Taking a long-term view of funding and its needs and pressures, often through an independent assessment, has avoided financial crises. The comparison with England's hand-to-mouth financial bungs and short-term initiatives could not be more striking.

Social care's zombie policy

The experience of other countries is important also in assessing arguments for using voluntary private insurance to fund social care. In their 2010 election manifesto, the Conservatives put forward a voluntary insurance plan whereby individuals could pay a premium of around £8,000 to protect their savings and assets from care home charges. The Adam Smith Institute has also argued that private insurers should be encouraged to develop new insurance and other financial products that people could choose to cover their costs of care (Butler and Saper, 2021). A former Cabinet minister once responsible for social care reform, Damian Green, has put forward the idea of a voluntary, insurance-funded care supplement that people could choose to pay to cover a higher-quality of accommodation or extra facilities and services (Green, 2020). The UK Parliament has debated a private member's bill put that would create a similar scheme to the one proposed in 2010, albeit with cover provided through a new state-backed company (UK Parliament, 2021). It is reported that Treasury officials are now working to encourage the industry, again, to develop fresh products on the back of the government's proposals to introduce, from 2023, a £86,000 cap on care costs, in the hope it will give insurers the certainty they need. According to the *Financial Times* (2021a), 'If insurance was available to cover expenses up to £86,000, it would help Boris

Johnson claim he was honouring the 2019 Conservative party manifesto pledge that "nobody needing care should be forced to sell their home to pay for it."'

This has been considered and dismissed by most independent reviews and commissions. For example, in 2011 the Dilnot Commission observed:

> We looked to see whether this was something that could be left to the private sector – as with areas such as house and car insurance. The problem is that there is currently too much uncertainty involved for the private sector to take on the full risk. There is uncertainty over how long people will live, uncertainty over changing care and support needs, uncertainty over costs, and uncertainty over wider changes that could affect care (such as medical advances or changes to the economy). These uncertainties have meant that the sector has struggled to design affordable and attractive products that people want to buy. No country in the world relies solely on private insurance for funding the whole cost of social care. (Dilnot, 2011)

Yet private insurance of social care is an idea that has proved remarkably difficult to kill off in England, hence its description here as a zombie policy. It's political resilience as a serious policy option owes much to the view that care is fundamentally the responsibility of the individuals and families, with the state offering only a basic safety net. Although the idea has been found wanting in the UK, to what extent has it been used by other countries to meet a significant share of care costs?

The overwhelming evidence is that it has not, except in very limited circumstances. Some countries have encouraged people to purchase long-term care insurance (LTCI) policies to close the gap in coverage and/or costs between public funding and the actual costs, but generally it plays a very minor role. In Europe, it is used only in France, Germany and Austria. Even in the USA, the poster boy for private insurance because of very limited public funding, the market was described over a decade ago as being 'in deep trouble', with rising premiums and more companies withdrawing from it (Gori et al, 2016). The Affordable Care Act ('Obamacare') has in effect converted some private insurance into mandatory public insurance through the Medicaid programme.

France is often highlighted as the only major country where private LTCI has expanded in recent years, encouraged by the way its public insurance scheme is structured and the low cost of premiums. Here, LTCI is often bundled with private health insurance. But the downside of low premiums is that the benefits are low too and usually cover only very high levels of need. So, despite more people having private LTCI in France than most other countries, it plays a minimal role in protecting people from care costs. Likewise, private LTCI policies have been available in Germany for many years but account for only 4 per cent of policies. Another review confirms that private LTCI plays a minor role in a few countries, but is generally less significant than voluntary insurance for health care. There is no evidence that any country uses private insurance as a substantive way of funding social care (Cylus et al, 2018). At best it will remain a niche or supplementary product, as in France.

The reasons why private insurance is rarely an effective or workable way of funding care have been well-documented (Comas-Herrera, 2012). Briefly, for the benefits to be meaningful, the premiums need to be high. This is, in part, because of the problems of adverse selection, whereby people with higher risks of needing to claim, such as those in later life or with existing illnesses, are much more likely to take out policies. As the Dilnot Commission pointed out, it is very hard for insurers to price such policies because of the inherent problems in aggregating likely needs and claims over 30 years or more. Indeed, the costs to insurers may well be prohibitive given the increasing numbers of people with multiple and chronic illness who are likely to make claims. Even if insurance cover were available, premiums are likely to be expensive, unaffordable and therefore regressive. Typically, premiums will be based on age and risk, not income. There is no widespread pooling of risk as there is with compulsory social insurance or universal coverage funded through taxation.

In England 'pre-funded' LTCI policies (those that are purchased well before the individual develops care needs) have not been available for some time. It was thought that the adoption of a cap on care costs proposed by the Dilnot Commission would encourage insurers to develop more affordable policies. But even the national voice of the UK insurance industry has doubted there will ever be a market for such policies, mostly because it would be hard to persuade younger people, indebted by the cost of student loans, mortgages and young families, to buy insurance for care (Association of British Insurers, 2014).

Overall, the extent of private household wealth in England (described in Chapter 2) raises some important questions for policy-makers in considering the role of private wealth in paying for care. The Johnson government's proposals to introduce a cap of £83,000 on private care costs from 2023 will blur the boundaries between private and public funding. The role of insurance has been resurrected once again and, although few believe pre-funded care insurance policies will re-emerge, there might be scope for other financial products to help with care costs. The mixed economy in the funding of care could be set to enter a new phase. It would be unwise to overlook the significant of private wealth in the future funding of care. This will be discussed in the final chapter.

6

Who cares?

A home is not a home but neither is it a hospital nor yet a hotel. What do we call the old people who live (and die) there … residents? Patients? Inmates? No word really suits. And who looks after them? Nurses? Not really since very few of them are qualified. As Mam pointed out early in her residency: "They're not nurses these. Most of them are just lasses."

Alan Bennett, *Untold Stories*

Care in the time of coronavirus

In 2021, COVID-19 swept through England's care services. The impact on people receiving care and support was profound, with over 27,000 'excess' deaths (those above the number that would usually be expected) in care homes and nearly 10,000 lives lost among those receiving care at home (Dunn et al, 2021). Visiting restrictions to limit the spread of the virus caused further anguish to care home residents and their families and friends. The high numbers of deaths among people with learning disabilities, people sectioned under the Mental Health Act and those from ethnic minority groups highlighted by independent researchers and the Care Quality Commission ought to attract more concern than it has. The pandemic also lifted the lid on the experience of the health and social care workforce and created new awareness of the experience of those working in care.

Before COVID-19 came, social care was not seen as a job like coal-mining or deep-sea fishing, where going to work might cost you your life. By December 2020, the virus had taken the lives of 469 care workers, twice the rate of all workers and even higher than health care workers, including doctors and nurses (ONS, 2021b). Levels of staff sickness nearly doubled over the course of the pandemic (Skills for Care, 2021). On the one hand, it has brought out the best in our care services, the way staff went beyond the call of duty in, for example, covering the work of colleagues who were sick or self-isolating, prioritising the protection of people they were caring for over their own needs and those of their own families. There were scores of stories of, for example, care workers who moved into their care homes to reduce the risks to residents (BBC News, 2020). But the worst aspects of working in social care were all too evident. Poor terms and conditions – low pay, zero-hours contracts, the absence of sick pay, reliance on agency staff moving from one home to another – caused staff to be an unwitting source of infection.

Care home manager Marlene Kelly offers a practical example of the dilemmas facing many care workers at the height of the coronavirus crisis:

> At the end of the day, with sickness you just find yourself thinking what can I do? I can't really stay out of work because if I stay out I'm just going to be paid statutory sick pay ... That doesn't pay your bills, that doesn't pay anything. And you find yourself struggling. (Health and Social Care Committee, 2020)

Her testimony illustrates the different experiences of staff working in social care compared with those working in the NHS:

> There was this amazing sign in a shop window saying 30 per cent off for all NHS employees. That is really demoralising, because we are making the same effort and doing the same work. There are people here who worked 14-hour days and went to the shops at the end of the evening, trying to provide for their family,

but were not given the opportunity to cut the line, because they did not wear an NHS badge.

For many care workers it was a harrowing time, captured in this testimony from someone who preferred to remain anonymous:

> It's actually been horrible because you don't know exactly what will become of you, you don't know what you are carrying within yourself, you don't know how long you can sustain without being infected. ... It's scary. You just live day by day and you just see how much your body is telling you. Most of the time I try as much as possible when I am [home] from work to ... stay away from [my children] which is ... not too nice.

In September 2021, Channel 4 broadcast *Help*, a powerful two-hour drama depicting a Liverpool care home ravaged by the virus (BBC News, 2021). Its central segment shows how Sarah, a relatively inexperienced care worker, finds herself working a 20-hour shift on her own, without support, no PPE and unable to get medical help for residents who are desperately ill and dying. It was a raw, moving drama, based on research from care homes throughout the country. More moving still was that so many care workers could see their own experience mirrored in the drama – 'Yes, that's what it was like.' COVID-19 has opened a new window into the world of care work.

The job of care

Ensuring that there are sufficient numbers of the right people, with the right skills and aptitude and supported and remunerated in a way that reflects the value of their work, is critical to a 21st-century system of social care that is fit for purpose.

In the world of work, and of public services, social care is big. Much is made of the NHS being in the top ten of the largest employers in the world, with 1.3 million people on its payroll. But social care is bigger, with 1.5 million people in England. They are mostly employed by 17,700 separate private or voluntary organisations (Skills for Care, 2021). It covers a disparate collection of roles, as Figure 6.1 shows, but is dominated by a vast army of care workers split fairly evenly between home care services and care homes.

There are 12 per cent more jobs now than in 2012, but numbers have fallen slightly since March 2021 due to the effects of COVID-19. It is becoming much harder to find people to do these jobs. Around 105,000 posts were vacant on any given day in 2019, an average vacancy rate of 6.8 per cent, compared

Figure 6.1: Individual job roles in adult social care

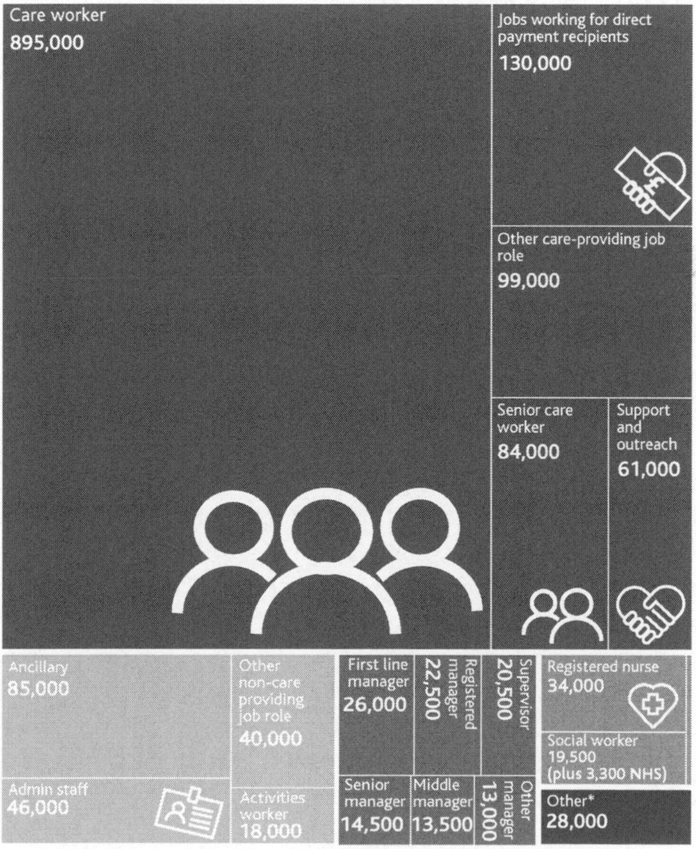

Occupational therapists **3,500 (plus 18,500 NHS)**

* 'Other' includes 11 job roles which were estimated to include fewer than 6,000 jobs each.

Source: Skills for Care (2021)

with 2.1 per cent for the economy as a whole. Employers are struggling to keep up as the number of jobs continues to grow, not helped by falling unemployment in the general economy. As competing employment sectors such as hospitality and tourism open up after the 2020 lockdown, the pressures are getting worse. By February 2022, the overall vacancy rate in the care sector had reached 9.5 per cent, but was much higher for care workers (11.8 per cent), registered managers (12.6 per cent) and registered nurses (17 per cent). The overall vacancy rate in London was noticeably higher, at 13 per cent (Skills for Care, 2022).

Although there has been much discussion about the problems that Brexit and recent changes to immigration policy have created for social care (discussed later), the underlying causes of today's serious workforce pressures long predate these changes. They are linked to the wider failure of governments over many years to reform social care and an over-concentration on how care is paid for rather than on who does the caring. Much of England's crisis in care is a crisis in workforce and stems from a failure to assess and plan workforce needs over many years.

The vast majority of hands-on care in hospitals, care homes and people's own homes is done by workers without a professional qualification. Just 5 per cent of social care jobs are in regulated professions. The largest of these is not, as one might expect, social work – 19,500 – but registered nurses – 34,000. Usually employed in nursing homes, where the clinical needs of residents are increasing, it is worrying that there are 30 per cent fewer nurses working in social care since 2012. This reflects a national and global shortage of nurses. It helps to explain the fragile state of the nursing home market in some parts of the country, such that the Care Quality Commission reports some homes cancelling their registration because they were unable to recruit nurses (Care Quality Commission, 2021). It might be surprising too that councils employ so few occupational therapists – 3,500 – given that they respond to between a third and a half of all referrals made to local councils and play a pivotal role in helping people to be independent and in need of less social care (Royal College of Occupational Therapists, 2021).

Whereas this 5 per cent of regulated professionals have received education and training to degree level, the qualification levels for the 95 per cent of the care workforce is rudimentary. The very basic requirement for care workers at entry level is the Care Certificate, introduced in 2015 and based on national occupational standards. Five years later, only 30 per cent of the workforce had completed it and 55 per cent had not even begun it. Progress on formal qualifications is no more encouraging: 56 per cent of the workforce (excluding those in the regulated professions) have no relevant care qualifications. Just 17 per cent had achieved NVQ (national vocational qualifications) at Level 3. This is not to say that care workers do not receive on-the-job training covering crucial aspects of their role, such as moving and handling, infection control and safeguarding, but even here the picture is patchy: only 56 per cent have received training on the safe handling of medication, on mental capacity and on deprivation of liberty rules. The contrast with the much more professionalised and qualified NHS could not be more vivid, even allowing for the longer, complex, science-based nature of health care professional training. Over 55 per cent of the NHS workforce belong to a regulated profession.

Particular mention must be made of the fastest growing role in social care – personal assistants (PAs) – who form the second largest group of staff in the workforce. They are employed directly by disabled people using a direct payment from their council to make their own care and support arrangements. For this group of workers, the numbers are heading in the right direction. There are now about 135,000 in PA roles, up 43 per cent since 2012 (Skills for Care, 2021). This does not include people who use their own money to employ a PA. They are recruited by individuals, not formal care organisations and most (58 per cent) are drawn from personal networks of friends and family who would not necessarily have considered working in social care.

With a big workforce comes a big pay bill: around £23 billion in 2019. More than two-thirds of the money spent on social care are on the wages and salaries of staff. But the bill should be bigger than it is. Social care services are blighted not only by low levels of training and qualification but low pay. It has the dubious distinction of having been defined as a low-pay industry by the Low Pay Commission (LPC) every year since its first report in 1998. The introduction of the national minimum wage (NMW) and later the national living wage (NLW) has helped to drive up pay levels, especially for the lowest paid, but there have been downsides. The 2.2 per cent increase in April 2021 is adding almost half a billion pounds to the pay bill, not covered by the extra funding to councils. It has become another cost pressure in the system (ADASS, 2021). The NLW has also narrowed the differentials with more senior roles. Instead of recognising greater skills and experience, care workers with five years or more experience are paid just 6 pence more per hour than those with less than one year of experience. This makes it next to impossible to offer care workers attractive career opportunities and training development. Another effect of the NMW/NLW has been to narrow the gap between social care and other low-paid jobs. In 2012–13, kitchen and catering assistants earned 53 pence less per hour on average than care workers, but this gap had reduced to 29 pence by 2020–21. Similarly, sales and retail assistants earned 13 pence per hour less than care workers in 2012–13, but, by 2020–21, they were earning 21 pence more per hour on average (ONS, 2021c). The NMW/NLW has not resolved the problem of low pay. The median hourly rate for care workers in March 2021 was £9.01, just 29 pence higher than the NLW. In April 2021, 35 per cent were being paid below the new rate of £8.91 per hour (Skills for Care, 2021b).

The combined impact of Brexit, the coronavirus and the furlough scheme, designed to help employers pay the wages of personnel unable to work during the pandemic, has seen escalating staff shortages in many other parts of the economy. There are now signs that social care is being overtaken by rising pay rates in retail, hospitality and other sectors in response to staff shortages. Many companies, such as Amazon, Tesco and John Lewis, are offering a joining bonus of £1,000 to attract new recruits (BBC News, 2021a). It is getting even harder to recruit people to care jobs.

Almost a quarter of care workers have zero-hours contracts, where the employer is not obliged to offer a minimum number of working hours. In home care services, this proportion rises to over half of the workforce, figures that have barely changed in recent years. About half of care staff work part-time, although people in managerial and professional roles were much more likely to work full-time.

There is a lot of churn among care jobs. Turnover rates have been rising steadily, with an overall rate of around 28 per cent, but most leavers find another job in the sector. Turnover is even higher among care workers, at 34 per cent. For registered nurses in social care, it is 38 per cent, over four times higher than their counterparts in the NHS. This is very bad news for the many people with care needs, who value continuity in their support instead of a sea of ever-changing faces. It also means that employers have higher recruitment costs, taking money that could otherwise be invested in training or better conditions of service.

Another area of vulnerability is the ageing of the workforce. Contrary to the experience of Alan Bennett's mum, most care workers are not 'just lasses' (Bennett, 2008). The average age is 44. Nearly everyone who works in social care – 91 per cent – is, over 25 years old, and over a quarter –27 per cent – are over 55 (compared with 21 per cent of the general population). That is 410,000 jobs that will have to be filled when they retire at some point in the next ten years. If anything, employers need to get much better at recruiting and retaining younger people.

Although the overall averages are grim, the numbers conceal some high spots. Just under a quarter of independent employers have a turnover rate of less than 10 per cent. Some employers are much more successful than others in recruiting and retaining staff. There is much evidence about the importance of culture, values and leadership, especially the key role of the registered manager, in the ability of a service to recruit and retain staff. There is a direct link to the quality of care: services rated as 'inadequate' or 'requires improvement' by the regulator are much more likely to have high turnover. And despite the high numbers of staff changing jobs, there is a solid core of experience in the workforce. The majority of staff – 79 per cent – had been working in social care for at least three years, with senior care workers having 11 years' experience on average.

Brexit and immigration

As in the NHS, many employers in social care have looked to ease their workforce problems by recruiting from other countries.

In 2021, a quarter of a million social care workers in England – 16 per cent of the social care workforce – came from abroad, compared with 8 per cent of the country's total workforce. Of these, 113,000 were from EU countries. Some parts of England have become much more reliant on non-British workers. In London, they represent 37 per cent of all care workers, and, in the South East, 23 per cent, whereas in Yorkshire and Humberside, it is just 7 per cent. The two most common nationalities of non-British care workers are Romanian and Polish, accounting for 22 per cent of the non-British workforce. One trend that has particular significance following the UK's departure from the EU and the introduction of new immigration rules is the proportion of registered nurses from EU countries doubling to 16 per cent since 2012, a worrying trend given high turnover and vacancy rates for this pivotal group of staff.

Since Brexit, workers from the EU have needed to obtain 'settled status' (the right to live and work in the UK) to continue to work here, unless they already have British citizenship. Another change has been the introduction of a points-based immigration system from January 2021. Under this, the job of 'care worker' was not included in the list of jobs deemed to be 'skilled'. In addition, most care jobs would have fallen foul of the minimum annual salary threshold of £20,489 required for admission to the UK unless they were included in the 'shortage occupation list' (Home Office, 2021). In short, it became impossible for people from other countries to become a care worker in the UK. So, there has been a sharp fall in the number of people arriving in the UK to take up social care jobs, making up just 1.8 per cent of new starters in the first quarter of 2021, compared with over 5 per cent during the same period in 2019 (although some of this reduction will have been due to temporary COVID-19 travel restrictions.) Fortunately, there are few signs of non-British care staff leaving the country since these changes.

Much has been made of the feared impact of the new immigration regime and Brexit on shrinking the social workforce, but the Migration Advisory Committee is surely right to say that the root cause of the workforce shortage in social care is not immigration controls, but the lack of competitive pay and conditions of service. Until those are improved significantly – and there is no sign of the government willing the means to do that – closing off overseas recruitment will only make it more difficult to plug workforce gaps. The impact will be felt most keenly in those parts of the country that have found it difficult to recruit from their existing population.

It is a measure of the growing concern about the workforce crisis during the pandemic that the government asked the Migration Advisory Committee to review the position and then on Christmas Eve 2021 accepted its recommendation that health and care workers should be added to the occupation shortage list for an initial period of 12 months (DHSC, 2021e). The value of this reprieve is limited. Workers from abroad will still need to earn at least £20,480 a year to qualify for a one-year visa, and it remains a complex and bureaucratic process (National Care Forum, 2022).

Another threat to the supply of care workers came from a new requirement that all care workers in care homes, but not in other care settings or the NHS, would be required to have full vaccination against COVID-19 by November 2021. The policy was quickly dubbed 'no jab, no job.' There are strong professional and medical arguments for such a policy. Care home residents are at much higher risk of infection and the complications that go with it. There are exemptions for those unable to have the vaccine for clinical reasons. But, as many very concerned care providers pointed out, the benefits of protecting residents from COVID-19 has to be balanced against the risks of poorer care from deteriorating levels of staffing. By the government's own assessment, mandatory vaccination could lead to the exodus of between 17,000 and 70,000 care staff who were unwilling or unable to be vaccinated (DHSC, 2021a).

Despite these worries, the government pressed ahead and planned to go further still by extending the policy to all regulated health and care settings by 1 April 2022. But, as concern mounted about the impact on overstretched hospital staffing, the government announced on 1 February that it planned to remove the requirement not only for NHS staff but social care as well. Compulsion was no longer considered balanced or proportionate with the lower risks from the Omicron variant of the virus. This was too late for the thousands of care workers who had already resigned or had their contracts terminated. No wonder the climbdown was greeted angrily by sector leaders, aggrieved that their concerns had been ignored and that care homes had been used as 'unwitting guinea pigs' in being expected to enforce 'a chaotic policy that is now considered obsolete' (Learner, 2022).

Women's work?

The single most striking characteristic of care work is that it is done overwhelmingly by women. Eighty-two per cent of paid care workers are female, compared with just 47 per cent in the general, economically active population. This goes for most kinds of jobs in the care sector, except for senior management roles, where it drops to 68 per cent. The same pattern can be found in most countries – in European Union countries it is even higher at 90 per cent (European Commission, 2021).

The majority of unpaid care is also provided by women, usually wives or partners and daughters. As we saw in Chapter 3, the economic value of their work, at £196 billion, completely dwarfs other elements of the social care pound. COVID-19 has swollen their ranks, with another 4.5 million people providing unpaid care because of the pandemic. 2.8 million of them are trying to hold down a paid job at the same time. The 9 million existing unpaid carers were doing more as well (Carers UK, 2020a). Unpaid carers are much less likely to be employed in paid work, however, contributing to the overall gender pay gap and gender pension gap. Their work is largely invisible.

Although governments have encouraged women to enter the labour market, they have assumed, as William Beveridge did when designing the welfare state in the 1940s, that women would continue to rock the cradle. Although female employment rates have risen since the 1970s, good child care facilities and formal care services have not kept pace. This helps to explain why women with children or other caring roles are more likely to be in part-time, low-paid and casualised jobs. The state provides even less support for unpaid carers than it used to, and satisfaction rates of unpaid carers with that support have fallen with it. There is abundant evidence that, while many carers choose to care and want to do so, for women especially, caring is bad for their income, their pensions and their overall health and wellbeing. And when it comes to the care needs that women themselves will have in later life, there is a double or even triple whammy: although female life expectancy is higher than men's, they are more likely to have poorer health and to live alone – because they live longer it is less likely they will have a spouse or partner to help them. So, more older women than older men might need long-term care, but are less able to access or afford it.

The enduring assumption that care is women's work has without doubt acted as a drag anchor on so many efforts to reform social care. Historically, there has been a tendency for society to devalue occupations that have developed traditionally as roles for women: care work is no exception. Political discussions about social care over the years have been punctuated periodically by calls for families to do more, recently expressed by former health Secretary Sajid Javid: "Government shouldn't own risks and responsibilities in life. We as citizens have to take some responsibility for our health too. We shouldn't always go first to the state. What kind of society would that be? Health – and social care – begins at home. Family first, then community, then the state" (Javid, 2021).

So, although social care is an overall force for good for society, in its current guise it contributes massively to gender inequalities. A strong argument for adequately funded, well-designed care services with good jobs and working conditions is that they would reduce these differences by making it easier for people to reconcile paid employment with unpaid caring roles. As Minouche Shafik has pointed out, it is no surprise that countries with the most generously funded care systems have the highest rates of female employment and the lowest gender inequality (Shafik, 2021). There is a strong argument that tackling gender inequality and reforming social care go hand in hand.

'I'm only a carer'

One of the remarkable aspects of the TV drama *Help*, discussed earlier, was the strength of the relationships between Sarah and the residents of the care home. The significance of those relationships should never be under-estimated.

Chapter 3 offered a reminder that people can receive a poor service yet express satisfaction with the experience because they had a good relationship with the social worker or care worker. The quality of that human connection is fundamental to people's experience of using social care and the outcome achieved. Often, it is the small things that make a big difference. Melanie Cairnduff, a senior care worker, explains:

> It is what I do for them. It is not what I do for the company I work for or for myself. It is seeing the people we look after smile every day, or when you are leaving they have a little grin on their face and they say thank you. That is what I do my job for. That is what I would say to anybody who wants to go into care. You have to not do it for the money. Obviously, the money helps because we all have bills to pay, but you have to do it because you want to make somebody else happy. You want to make them have the best life they possibly can.
>
> Most of my work is long-term care and building relationships and all the tiny things, like where the soap is, in someone's home, need to be learned so I can support them – I like working with people like this.
>
> If you know what they like – how they have the curtains drawn, their favourite breakfast cereal and if you really know your clients and build relationships, that's what I really enjoy.
>
> You make a difference. You might be the only person they see in a day. (Health and Social Care Committee, 2020)

Raina Summerson, who has worked her way up from care worker to chief executive of a large care organisation, explains the emotional investment of carers in their work:

> That means they are emotionally affected. They are the ones who have to shut the door and walk away up the garden path, leaving people when they know

they did not really get the time they needed. They may have missed out on the preventive services that were there 10 or 15 years ago. That affects their morale and job satisfaction, and that affects retention. No matter what training or pay you give them, if that is their experience every day, it is not going to change. (Health and Social Care Committee, 2020)

The social care system has come to be heavily dependent on the intrinsic job satisfaction and altruism of care workers instead of financial reward, recognition, and investment in education, skills and training. The raw metrics of pay, turnover and casualisation paint a grim picture of how much we expect from people who work in social care for so little by way of pay and working conditions. Instead, employers rely on what workforce researcher Eleanor Johnson describes as the 'moral currencies of hugs and thank yous' (Johnson, 2015). A belief in the intrinsic value of care work and rewarding relationships with service users are known to be major factors that encourage people to enter and remain in the workforce (Chambers et al, 2019). The fulfilling nature of care work is described by the CEO of one care company, in a video for new staff, as a 'second pay cheque'. The government's 'Made with Care' recruitment campaign variously describes social care jobs as 'rewarding', 'making a difference every day through patient, commitment and compassion' and offering an opportunity to 'find fulfilment' (DHSC, 2022b). 'Kindness has its own reward' is used as a recruitment strapline by a major care home company.

It ought to be a cause of national embarrassment that the emotional value of caring is exploited in order to maintain a culture of low pay and poor working conditions. When people who work in social care say, 'I'm only a carer', it shows how much the low status of care work is routinely internalised by those who do it. Camilla Cavendish captures it well:

The paradox is that some of the lowest paid care workers are those who we expect to work the most independently, walking into the homes of strangers, and having to tackle what they find there, without any direct supervision. This requires a high level of maturity and resilience. Calling this 'basic' care does not reflect the fact that getting it right is a deeply skilled task. (Department of Health, 2013)

When things go wrong, it is too easy for the care worker to take the rap when they are being expected to do too much. Jonathan, whose mother lived in residential care, explains:

I talked about some of the amazing care my mum received, but it is often very much on the basis of the personal contribution that care workers put in. In even the very best of homes you can see how they are stretched. You can see how the staff are not supported. I brushed over some of the mistakes in the first care home, but it is overworked and under-recognised staff who make mistakes like putting the wrong 'Do not resuscitate' order on the wrong file, which is what happened in my situation. (Health and Social Care Committee, 2021a)

Our thinking about the people who do care work, whether paid or unpaid, can be coloured also by different views about what we mean by this small word 'care', which, as Madeleine Bunting points out in *Labour of Love*, has 'a large empire of meanings' (Bunting, 2020). It is central to our experience of growing up, as parents and grandparents bring up children, roles that may be reversed later on. Care is threaded through our personal friendships, romantic love and our networks of neighbours and friends. For millions of people, it is something they are paid to do, involving the application of professional skill as well as interpersonal relationships, as part of a sector or an industry – the fastest growing form of employment in most wealthy countries. It can be formal and informal, paid and unpaid.

In her book *An Extra Pair of Hands*, author Kate Mosse movingly describes her experience of caring for both her parents and her mother-in-law over a number of years. As she says of the term 'care':

It's a tricky word. It's a noun freighted with meaning and requiring qualification. It brings with it a hint of transaction, of an inequality, which is all the more uncomfortable if you're caring for someone you love. By using it, however accurate it might be in terms of the day-to-day realities, there's a risk that it redefines a partnership, a balanced give-and-take relationship, and turns it into an obligation: carer and patient, carer and client. One is active, the other passive, whereas ever carer knows there's nearly always some kind of reciprocity even in the darkest hours. You are still you, and they are still they. (Mosse, 2021)

Rigid demarcations between people who do the caring and those who receive it overlook not only the power of relationships but the importance of reciprocity and interdependence that have come up time and time again in the many conversations I have had in the writing of this book. Much of the discussion about people who work in social care is couched in the industrialised language of workforce, recruitment, retention and turnover. It sounds more like Soviet plans for tractor production instead of the intensely personal and individual experiences of carers and cared-for that has always been the defining feature of good care and support. It is as though the problem is just about the quantity of people, as units of labour, rather than the quality of the relationships with those they work with.

A small and personal example. When my father died, after spending the last four years of life in a care home, I was moved by the number of messages I received from members of staff, and by conversations I have had with some of them since. They described what he had contributed to their lives, and those of his fellow residents. They ranged from making bird tables for the garden, helping new residents settle in or putting a smile on the face of staff during a stressful day. The reality that care involves reciprocity, about relationships rather than the receipt of a service, is at the heart of vision developed by the #SocialCareFuture movement that says, 'When organised well, social care helps to weave the web of relationships and support in our local communities that we can draw on to live our lives in the way that we want to, with meaning, purpose and connection, whatever our age or stage of life' (Crowther and Quinton, 2021).

The etymology of the term 'care' reflects two quite different meanings. The first involves purposeful activity to help someone's health and welfare – caring *for* someone. The second is more about an attitude of concern or empathy for a particular person or group of people – caring *about* someone. Good social care and professional social work ought to embrace both – arguably care workers should care *for* people because they care *about* them. Social workers, for example, as a condition of their registration are expected to uphold professional standards based on valuing the individual and upholding their human rights, views, wishes and feelings (Social Work England, 2019). Social care workers in England are not required to be registered, unlike those in other parts of the UK, so there is no comparable statement of values or conduct, although the basic induction programme for new staff, the Care Certificate, is based on standards that include these values.

The distinction between caring *for* and caring *about* someone is not straightforward, but it goes to the heart of social care's purpose. Where the balance between the two falls will depend on the myriad variety of needs, expectations and preferences among the hundreds of thousands of people who draw on care and support. As described in Chapter 1, there are many disabled people for whom 'caring for' is synonymous with a traditional mindset that sees them as dependent and vulnerable, as passive recipients of traditional services in which power sits with professionals and organisations. Acts of care are acts of control, for example, where Jennifer Pearl, who needs help because of a spinal tumour, has to go to bed at 8 o'clock every night because that was the latest time the agency can offer (Pearl, 2021). In contrast, good support should be emancipatory, helping to remove the barriers that make it hard for people to go out and pursue friendships, leisure activities and ordinary acts of living that most people take for granted. Caring *about* someone involves an individual and collective commitment to upholding their rights as equal citizens. This includes offering people real choices in how the support they need is tailored to their particular circumstances, rather than 'one size fits all.' On the other hand, neither should we underestimate the sheer number of people for whom being 'cared for' is vitally important. For almost three-quarters of older people and nearly a third of working-age people receiving long-term care, the need for personal care is the main one. Projections of future needs suggest that more of us will need physical and personal care in the years ahead.

These reflections on what we mean by the term 'care' are important because much of the policy thinking about social care over the years has been deeply imbued with *a priori* beliefs about what care is and who should do it. Since 1948, the social care system in all parts of the UK has operated on an implicit presumption that families should normally be responsible for looking after their disabled and older relatives, and, where they cannot, it can be provided by those whose Alan Bennett's mum described as 'just lasses'. The professional contribution to such care is supplemental, such as a visiting GP or district nurse. In contrast, health care is seen as requiring a high-skill, professional and paid workforce. These views reflect and reinforce the perception that care work, unlike health care work, is unskilled. Arguably, this perception belongs to the same anachronistic mindset that objects to nursing becoming a graduate profession because nurses would become, in the colloquialism, 'too posh to wash'. But low pay does not mean low skill. Camilla Cavendish, who reviewed the work of unqualified workers in health and social care in 2014, was unequivocal:

> Helping an elderly person to eat and swallow, bathing someone with dignity and without hurting them, communicating with someone with early onset dementia; doing these things with intelligent kindness, dignity, care and respect requires skill. Doing so alone in the home of a stranger, when the district nurse has left no notes, and you are only being paid to be there for 30 minutes, requires considerable maturity and resilience. (Department of Health, 2013)

The professional and the personal

Does that mean the answer is a professionally qualified and regulated workforce? England is now the only part of the UK that does not require its workers to be registered with a national body charged with regulating and upholding standards, a key milestone towards the professionalisation of the workforce. Not everyone agrees this is a good thing. As noted earlier, the fastest growing part of the care workforce is that of personal assistants, who are employed directly by disabled people, using their direct payments, with control over who they choose to employ and what they want them to do by way of support. There is no requirement to screen or vet these PAs for criminal convictions or any other contraindications that might prevent them getting a job in a formally regulated service such as a care home. Trade unions representing care workers have argued that the growth of this unregulated workforce will place people at risk of exploitation and abuse and for PAs it will mean lower pay, less training and poorer conditions of service. As yet, there appears to be no evidence of greater referrals for suspected abuse where PAs are employed. On the contrary, although compared with the social care workforce, fewer PAs have a care qualification, they are more experienced, are paid more, stay in the role longer and are less likely to be on a zero-hours contract (Skills for Care, 2021a).

The risks of employing someone without the checks and safeguards required in regulated services can be greatly mitigated by the right approach to recruitment and support (Davey, 2020). Against those risks should be balanced the overwhelming popularity of direct payments with those who use them. Baroness Jane Campbell, a lifelong campaigner for disability rights and champion of direct payments, offers a crisp summary:

> We are aware of the risk and believe it has to be weighed against the drawbacks of compulsory registration – increased bureaucracy, additional expense and loss of control in our lives. For example, I have employed two individuals with criminal convictions of a kind that would prevent them registering and so make it impossible for me to employ them. Not only were they extremely good PAs, but I could give them employment at a time when their job prospects were gloomy. We assisted

each other, overcoming the social barriers that stood in our way. It was my calculated risk that took us both on this successful journey.

Many direct payments users will tell you that people who have no formal care training often make the best PAs. This is because they bring no preconceived ideas about how people should be cared for. Instead, they respond to the training from their employer, the person receiving direct payments. (Campbell, 2006)

Jane has regaled many an audience with her tale of how an applicant for a personal assistant job she liked had served time for being an armed robbery getaway driver and was a past associate of the Kray twins. She gave him the job and he turned out to be a great driver and one of the best personal assistants she has ever employed (Brindle, 2008).

A quantum of care

Looking to the future it is clear that we will need many more people to do care work. The latest estimates are staggering. By 2030, less than a decade away, it is estimated that 627,000 extra social care staff will be needed to improve services and meet need. This is a 55 per cent growth over the next decade and four times greater than the increases of the last ten years (Rocks et al, 2021). From a starting point of 104,000 vacancies and rising, this raises huge questions about who will fill these jobs, especially when the NHS also will need many more staff. As discussed earlier, there are immediate and short-term threats to the supply of care workers because of Brexit, the new immigration system and the consequences of mandatory vaccination of care home staff. But it is not just about numbers; it is about the nature of the work people are expected to do. It is not always appreciated how much more complex and demanding social care and social work has already become over the years.

Although social work is a relatively tiny slice of the workforce pie, the duties and demands placed on social workers bear no recognition to the profession I joined over four decades ago. Dealing with situations that are often complex and intractable, social workers have important legal powers to ensure that people's human rights and freedoms are protected. Sometimes, these must be balanced with the protection of the public, for example where someone with acute and serious mental illness has to be deprived of the freedom in order to ensure they can have essential treatment or are prevented from harming others.

When I began my social work career in the late 1970s, the possibility that parents might harm their children was not well established: my initial social work training covered 'non-accidental injury', focusing on physical harm. The extent of emotional and sexual abuse had yet to be appreciated. That older and disabled people might also be at risk of neglect, abuse and exploitation was further down the line. Not until the 1980s were councils and the social workers they employed given formal statutory powers to protect and safeguard adults.

More recently, new kinds of abuse, such as human slavery, forced marriages and female genital mutilation have added another layer to the complex judgements that social workers are expected to make. Social workers have become managers of risk. The concern to safeguard and protect people's rights and best interests has thrown up a new socio-legal concept of 'social care detentions'. These affect as many as 300,000 people without mental capacity, often those with dementia, neurological disorders or learning disabilities, who are deemed to have been deprived of their liberty and thus require legal protection. This has spawned a host of professional, legal and ethical dilemmas for practitioners and managers (Series, 2022). Grappling with these responsibilities while helping people to lead good lives and protecting their human rights is possible, but challenging (James et al 2019).

We expect more too of care workers, without the benefit of a professional qualification or training. Any seasoned social care professional will confirm that the level of need met in different care settings has escalated dramatically in the last three decades. Home care workers are now helping people with tasks, such as medication, dressings and managing continence, that previously would have been done by a district nurse. Residential care homes now cater for people with significant health care needs that previously would have been met in nursing homes. And nursing homes are routinely attending to very specialist and complex needs, often involving palliative and end-of-life care, that once would have been provided in a hospital or hospice. It is not just that more people need care, but that more people are needing more care. This is a direct consequence of the trends described in Chapter 2, namely, the greater complexity and acuity of needs arising from comorbidity, frailty and dementia, along with the gradual shift of responsibilities from the NHS to social care. It is the people who do care work who have borne the direct and personal consequences of these changes. As with the drift towards outsourced services, it as though social care services have sleepwalked into a situation where the heavy-lifting work of care, literally as well as metaphorically, is done by some of the least qualified, lowest paid and undervalued part of the workforce. In the history of social care and social work, we have never expected so much from so few. The trend shows no sign of abating. In the 20 years to 2035, there will be 127 per cent more over-85-year-olds with very high levels of care need. For people with dementia and at least two other illnesses, that increase exceeds 200 per cent (Kingston et al, 2018a).

These trends have big implications for the care workforce of the future, and not simply that we need more people to provide the higher volumes of support that needs to be delivered. The workforce of the future will require new skills and knowledge, as well as refreshing and updating their existing skills. This includes, for example, the use of digital technology and new policies and legislation (the introduction of Liberty Protection Safeguards to replace the existing Deprivation of Liberty safeguards is a case in point). More opportunities for professional and skills development and better supervision and support will be needed. There are question marks over the current demarcation between professionally qualified social workers educated to degree level, and social care workers whose access to training and education has usually been limited to vocational qualifications. This hard division will become increasingly inappropriate as the acuity and complexity of needs in all care settings continues to rise. This will apply not only to qualifications and training but also pay, support and supervision and opportunities for career progression. Finally, because more people will have clinical as well as care and support needs, or have other issues requiring multi-agency responses, care workers will need to develop their existing skills and work more closely with health and care staff from other disciplines, for example GPs and district nurses and hospital discharge specialists, so that people get joined-up, coordinated care. The boundaries between clinical and care roles in care homes and home care services are set to become even more blurred with the expansion of important initiatives such as enhanced health care in care homes (NHS England, 2020a).

From policy neglect to a people plan

One of the most conspicuous failures of successive governments in sorting out social care has been the neglect of its workforce in the face of mounting pressures from recruitment, retention and shortages of staff. These have been long in the making and are well recognised. The last workforce strategy was published in 2009 and is available only in the National Archives. It is so dated that some of the organisations assigned responsibilities in the document no longer exist. In 2018, the National Audit Office warned that the government must 'act quickly' to develop a workforce strategy to address the immediate challenges and set out how future workforce needs and numbers will be met (NAO, 2018). The government continues to resist calls from over 100 health and care organisations to produce biannual projections of workforce needs (Royal College of Physicians, 2022).

It is no wonder that social care was so ill-equipped when COVID-19 came. The poor pay and working conditions and job insecurity it highlighted should really have come as no surprise. After all, the main attraction of having most services delivered by independent organisations is that staff can be employed more cheaply than in the public sector. Much of the funding problem in social care has been exported to the pay packets and precarious employment arrangements of hundreds of thousands of care workers. It has taken a global pandemic to teach us that many of the workers we relied on the most – care workers, hospital porters and cleaners, delivery drivers, refuse collectors, for example – are paid and valued the least.

Unlike the NHS, with its 'People Plan' published in 2020 (NHS, 2020), social care still does not have a workforce strategy. The Westminster government has repeatedly declined to introduce mandatory registration of social care workers, unlike every other part of the UK. It is surely time to reconsider this anomaly as the centrepiece of wider reforms to raise the status of social care and improve standards as well as boost public confidence and awareness. The lack of investment in training and education is another deficit. The body responsible for education and training in the NHS, Health Education England, has an annual budget of £40 billion, whereas the closest equivalent for social care is £30 million, which works out at £14 per employee. Even allowing for the complexity and science-based nature of key NHS occupations, that is an enormous disparity (Humphries and Timmins, 2021). Workforce planning and development is in effect delegated to a registered charity. While that charity, Skills for Care, punches well above its weight in activity and influence, in other parts of the UK, the responsibility sits with a statutory body. This catalogue of policy neglect has helped to create a new and growing crisis of care in which lack of people joins lack of money in threatening the essential support and services that so many of us need.

In fairness, the government has recognised some of the problems and found some new money to address them. Its 'Build Back Better' proposals for health and social care published in September 2021, included a new workforce-development fund of £500m over three years to help professionalise the workforce and create 'hundreds of thousands of training places and certifications for our care workers.' (HM Government, 2021a). That works out roughly at £111 per employee per year. The White Paper 'People at the Heart of Care' sets out a list of actions to improve recruitment and support, including more financial help for providers. These measures are welcome but fall well short in terms of ambition and resources. The government's own impact assessment of its workforce proposals is silent on the matter of pay, even though this is frequently cited by employers as one of the biggest obstacles to recruitment (DHSC, 2022).

Instead of a collection of ad hoc initiatives, what is urgently needed is a comprehensive strategy, or People Plan, with some bold and imaginative thinking. This should:

- set out some steps in the short-term to halt the worsening crisis of turnover and shortages;
- a forward-plan to secure more care workers for the future and know where they will come from;
- establish mandatory professional registration for all social care workers in regulated services;
- in the longer term, lay the foundations for care work as a popular and valued career, with a well-paid and well-trained portfolio of jobs and roles.

There are plenty of ideas that the architects of a new people plan for social care could draw on. The most obvious and urgent starting point is to pay care workers a decent wage. An immediate first step could be to pay care workers a loyalty bonus of, say, £500 or £1,000 to say thank you and help staunch the flow of people leaving their jobs, as Wales, Scotland and Northern Ireland have done already. This was recommended by the task force established by the government to support social care during COVID-19 (DHSC, 2020a). A next step would be to raise average pay levels to at least 5 per cent above the NLW. This would help towards parity with the NHS. Pay progression could be improved further by linking care worker salaries with the pay bands for health care assistants under the NHS 'Agenda for Change' pay structure, as Scotland has already begun to do (Scottish Government, 2021a). This will not be cheap – lifting pay beyond the NLW alone would cost £3.9 billion a year by 2023–24 – but many of the higher pay costs would be returned to the public purse via higher tax receipts, lower benefit claims and the multiplier effect of care workers spending more in their local economy.

These early measures could help to turn around the system's dangerous over-reliance on the altruism of care workers as well as the diminishing supply of cheap labour at the expense of decent pay, training and support. But the roots of the current crisis in social care staffing run deeper. Higher pay is just a beginning – necessary but not sufficient. Action is also needed to improve the status of care work and offer people much more attractive career options. This could be based on a much clearer understanding of the needs, views and motivations of people who work in social care, perhaps based on something similar to the annual NHS Staff Survey in which everyone working in the NHS is invited to take part.

Tackling the workforce crisis is not all down to the government, but it does have a pivotal role to play. This is to set a national framework and strategy, ensuring that resources are available and aligning the various levers of policy and regulation. These include employment, economic and migration policies. And by addressing the wildly different levels of workforce investment in social care compared with the NHS. When the government has fulfilled its obligations, it is then down to local employers, supported by the councils that commission from them, to plan and work together to recruit, retain and support their local workforce. The scale of the staffing shortfall and increasing competitiveness of local labour markets requires employers, large and small, and even individuals employing their own personal assistants, to be ever more imaginative in how they attract the right people, use them wisely, invest in their development – and keep them.

Much can be learned from employers who have bucked the trend with turnover rates of less than 10 per cent. When asked what contributed to their success, investing in learning and development was top of the list (94 per cent), followed by embedding the values of the organisation (92 per cent), celebrating the achievements of both the organisation and the individual (86 per cent) and involving colleagues in decision-making (81 per cent). Values-based recruitment, compared with traditional recruitment, was associated with lower sickness rates, better skill development and higher performance in the job. Technology can help too. The Care Friends app, developed by recruitment guru Neil Eastwood, is making it easier for existing care workers to refer people they know for jobs. This has led to more people being recruited, and people who perform better and stay in post longer than those recruited through traditional internet boards (Skills for Care, 2021c). Skills for Care is using data science and machine learning to identify more accurately the factors associated with staff turnover. In many places, technology is beginning to ease the demands on care staff, improving both productivity and the quality of care. Examples include the use of smartphones, alarm systems, sensors, and GPS monitors and companionship robots. Comprehensive technologies, such as self-sufficient smart homes, can enhance – but not replace – the work of carers.

There are lots of opportunities to create really attractive and properly paid career pathways instead of the very limited opportunities and pay differentials currently available. Many care workers have skills and experience that would make a great foundation for professional training to become a registered nurse, social worker or occupational therapist, or even fill jobs in care commissioning or related sectors like supported housing and the voluntary sector. There are obvious potential bridges with NHS roles, such as health care assistants or nurse associates. There are opportunities to think about new kinds of hybrid roles in areas such as reablement and rehabilitation, digital technology and extra-care housing. Designing these new opportunities and career pathways would need a big expansion of training and education options at different levels and with a menu of affordable and sometimes part-time routes instead of the rigidity of a three-year full-time degree. These can be designed around a range of existing jobs and roles as well as new ones. PA roles could be included, building on the success and popularity of this role by offering a more formal approach to training and support and designing links to professional training for those who wish to develop their careers. This would make PA jobs even more attractive without undermining the freedom of people with direct payments to choose who they employ or risk over-professionalising a role that is working well for so many people.

There are so many ways in which a career in care could be reimagined as a career worth having, a career that belongs in a different league to supermarket shelf stackers, bar staff and cleaners.

England is not alone in experiencing problems with recruiting sufficient numbers of people with the right skills. Low pay, limited training and casualised employment arrangements are common in OECD countries (OECD, 2020a). It is hard to find one country that is leading the way in finding solutions, but there are plenty of examples we could learn from, especially about how the synergies between jobs in health and social care could be exploited to raise the status and skills of care work. The most well-known example is the Buurtzorg model, in which qualified nurses provide a mixture of health and care support through self-organised teams that promote autonomy and job satisfaction. In Denmark, there is an integrated training system for health and social care staff that provides degree-level qualifications to unqualified workers. It involves placements in a variety of care settings, such as hospitals, care homes and home care. Its multidisciplinary approach encourages mutual understanding of different roles and flexibility of roles. Norway introduced a 'Men in Health' recruitment programme to attract unemployed men aged 26 to 55 to the health and care sector. Japan increased its care workforce by 20 per cent between 2011 and 2015 through financial support for training, directed particularly at students and returning workers. Sweden is creating more permanent care jobs. Germany is raising pay levels (Hemmings, 2021). Closer to home, the Leeds Health and Social Care Academy is a joint venture between the NHS, local government and universities that takes a 'one workforce' approach to train, empower and support all staff across all health and care staff in the city (Leeds Health and Care Academy, 2021).

There are a couple of upgrades to the governance of the social care workforce that could also help. The first is to beef-up the status of Skills for Care by making it an executive agency with lead responsibility for developing a people plan, building on the strength of its existing networks of relationships with employers. It could also take on the responsibility, on behalf of the government, of conducting detailed projections of the future supply and demand for particular job roles so that employment gaps can be anticipated and prepared for. The second upgrade is to give the new Integrated Care Systems oversight of their local health care workforce planning and development, working in partnership with employers, councils and national skills bodies. Although some might see this as unhelpful incursion by the NHS into social care, its purpose would be developmental rather than controlling. The objective should be to ensure that NHS organisations (hospitals in particular) and their social care partners are working together to boost their local workforce rather than competing with each other for scarce staff such as registered nurses.

In conclusion, there can be no meaningful reform of social care without a reimagining of the nature of care and how we recognise, reward and support those who provide it, whether as paid employees or as unpaid family carers. This is not simply about how we 'fix the workforce' by paying people more or providing more training, important as those are. It raises fundamental questions about the social contract between the state, individuals and families established in the simpler times of the 1940s. In its uncodified form, women largely stayed at home and looked after their children and sometimes their parents as well. In return, the state would provide a retirement pension, family allowance and free education and child care. It is a social contract that is now completely unworkable, unfair and ineffective, up-ended by 70 years of rapid changes in society, demography and changing family structures. Nowhere is that more obvious than in the operation of an adult social care system that remains rooted in the assumptions of the 1940s and places the heaviest burdens of care on those ill-equipped and supported to carry it. At the heart of a better social care system must be a new social contract between individuals, families and the state. This will be central to the proposals set out in the final chapter.

7

A 1948 moment? The politics and process of reform

> A revolutionary moment in the world's history
> is a time for revolution not a time for patching.
> William Beveridge, 1942

A new Beveridge?

COVID-19 has laid bare more than just the many deep-seated problems of England's social care system that have defied the attempts of every government since the 1990s to tackle. Many of these problems date back to the absence of social care from the welfare state settlement after the Second World War. COVID-19 has also heralded sweeping changes in how we lead our lives, how we work, shop and engage with friends, families and wider social networks. In many places, it has led to a surge in community spirit, in neighbourliness and volunteering. Necessity demanded that councils work in different, more productive ways with their partners in private, voluntary, community and social enterprise sectors. The rapidity of some of these shifts in working practices and decision-making, compared with the normally placid pace of policy-making, brings to mind Lenin's dictum that 'there are decades where nothing happens; and there are weeks where decades happen.'

This renewed sense of social solidarity and the heightened exposure of the public to the realities about social care, as well as the inequalities in wider society revealed by the pandemic.

have together prompted debate as to whether the current crisis offers the opportunity for a 'new Beveridge', a 21st-century version of that seminal report that was to lay the foundations of the post-war British welfare state. The impact of COVID-19 has boosted the argument that fundamental changes can no longer be postponed and that there is now an unmissable opportunity to grasp the nettle of reform. The phrase 'Build Back Better' has been widely used, here and in the USA, to convey a sense of the large-scale renewal and reconstruction that is needed as the country emerges from the pandemic. As development and globalisation expert Ian Goldin observes, the pandemic came on top of other escalating crises around the world. He points to those in climate change, geopolitics and social inequalities; changes that are creating immense strains in many societies. His clarion call is for radical changes, rather than a return to 'business as usual':

> COVID-19 has created a pivotal moment. Everything hangs in the balance. The pandemic compressed into a year trends that otherwise would have taken decades to emerge. It has brought us to an inflection point in history. By seizing this historic moment, we can turn the tide to shape our individual and collective destiny, and in so doing we would rescue humanity from catastrophe and create a better world. (Goldin, 2021)

It was a Labour government that created the welfare state, but over 75 years later, it is a Conservative one that is presiding over 'the biggest expansion of state intervention in economic and social life that has ever been witnessed since' (Coats, 2020). Compared with the years of financial austerity from 2010, the sudden switch to 'Big State' levels of spending invited some to wonder whether social care's time had now come. In April 2021, 26 national leaders and politicians wrote to the prime minister calling for 'a 1948 moment' for adult social care, to establish a long-term and sustainable future that will benefit all citizens and the economy (Care England, 2021). Inspired by the spirit of the social solidarity of the first COVID-19 lockdown in 2020, historian Peter Hennessy has set out a 'new Beveridge' manifesto, with social care reform at the top of his list of five shared 'tasks' for a new post-COVID settlement (Hennessy, 2022). So, are we now on the cusp of a Beveridge moment for social care? Or will COVID-19, as others have opined, be another crisis of which the political effects will quickly wash away? (Burchardt, 2020).

There are some obvious parallels between the country's experiences in the Second World War and the pandemic. Both involved massive loss of life and huge collective sacrifice, with profound social and economic impacts on people's lives. The UK economy crashed by 10 per cent in 2020, a much sharper downturn than most other advanced economies and said to be the biggest recession since the Great Frost of 1709. Higher government spending on the costs of COVID-19 caused the national debt to soar to more than 100 per cent of GDP. It was even higher in the war-ravaged 1940s, when the country was afflicted by widespread shortages of food, fuel and housing and both a balance of payments and a sterling crisis. After years of privation and misery, it was no wonder that William Beveridge's 1942 blueprint to tackle the 'five giant evils' of 'want, disease, ignorance, squalor and idleness' captured the national mood.

The Beveridge Report sold 100,000 copies within a month of publication, and eventually 635,000; figures that put it on a par with bestselling works of fiction. As Peter Hennessy observes, 'there has never been an official report like it' (Hennessy, 2006). A Gallup survey in 1943 showed that 19 out of 20 people knew about the report and, more to the point, supported it. A full 86 per cent were in favour of its plans for free health care, family allowances and social security, a major house-building programme and full employment. Free health care achieved 88 per cent. Public support was overwhelming and sufficient to overcome the resistance of the Treasury, which thought the plans were unaffordable. The result of the 1945 general election put the outcome in no doubt.

So it was that, in the teeth of a raging economic crisis and bankrupt public finances, the welfare state, inspired by the Beveridge Report, rose from the ashes of war. But, for reasons discussed in Chapter 2, it did not include social care within its remit other than with the barest of safety nets, the National Assistance Act 1948.

The omens for a new settlement akin to the 1940s are not encouraging. The government's 'Build Back Better' plan for health and social care had an eyebrow-raising proposal to put up National Insurance and earmark, or hypothecate, the proceeds for the NHS and social care. Initially, most of the new money raised will go towards tackling the NHS waiting list backlogs, burgeoning because of COVID-19. Later, it will be used to fund a cap on care costs. As discussed in Chapter 4, similar proposals were accepted by the coalition government before being abandoned by the Cameron government after the 2015 election. It is designed to sort out one particular problem affecting a relatively small proportion of people with care and support needs.

The principles behind the Johnson government's proposals for social care have been welcomed, but few believe that they offer the long-term plan that social care so badly needs. Furthermore, any attempt to 'build back better' on the fragile foundations of the current social care system are unlikely to end well. Referring to the need to 'turbo-charge' the transformation of social care, Caroline Abrahams, speaking for the Care and Support Alliance, likened the White Paper 'People at the Heart of Care' to 'an underpowered saloon car' rather than a 'formula one vehicle' (Care and Support Alliance, 2021; DHSC, 2021c). As things stand, to paraphrase Beveridge, this bears scant resemblance to a revolutionary moment but instead takes us back to where we were in 2015 when similar, but more generous, plans had been legislated for and funding agreed. Many years on, patching, not fundamental reform remains the order of the day.

Widespread news reporting of the impact of COVID-19 on care homes has helped to raise the public's awareness of social care. When asked in September 2021 what were the biggest issues facing the country, 12 per cent of the British public spontaneously mentioned social care (Ipsos Mori, 2021a). In the long history of the monthly Ipsos opinion poll, this is a sharp increase on previous ratings. In recent times, the top issues have been dominated by COVID-19, the NHS, the economy and Brexit, with social care rarely making it into the top ten issues of concern. At the height of the pandemic in 2020, it barely registered at all. So, while COVID-19 may have nudged social care out of the shadows, this is a long way off the stratospheric levels of public awareness and support enjoyed by the Beveridge Report in the 1940s.

Another difference is that, despite the economic shock of COVID-19, the economy looks to be bouncing back much more quickly than anticipated, much faster than after the 2008 recession. Because of buoyant tax receipts and tax increases, the prospects for public finances had, in the words of the independent Institute for Fiscal Studies, 'improved hugely' and the budget deficit seems likely to be eliminated by 2023, the first time since the turn of the millennium (Emmerson and Stockton, 2021). There remain considerable risks and uncertainties about prospects for inflation and interest rates and the impact of soaring energy prices on national and household finances, together with the future trajectory of COVID-19, including the emergent of new variants and the medium- to longer-term effects of vaccination. It does look, however, as though the combined social and economic repercussions of COVID-19 will be nothing like the profound and lasting devastation the country faced after the war. Indeed, that our economic circumstances are much better than they were in 1948 makes it much harder to water-down plans for better social care on grounds of unaffordability.

The analogy with Beveridge is further strained by the unequal impact of COVID-19 on lives and livelihoods. The universal experience of total war, and the depression of the 1930s that preceded it, saw many millions experience poverty, unemployment and economic privations and led to a national appetite for a more equal society after 1945. In contrast, COVID-19 has impacted disproportionately on people with low or no incomes, those in deprived neighbourhoods, in overcrowded housing and from black and ethnic minority groups. Far from being a great leveller, COVID-19 has deepened inequalities COVID(Bambra et al, 2021).

For all these reasons, the prospects for a new Beveridge, including a new settlement for social care, are not auspicious. While there are powerful arguments that the opportunities created by the COVID-19 crisis should not be allowed to go to waste, today's circumstances are very different from the post-war world and there is no obvious contender to inherit William Beveridge's mantle.

So, if the economic and social shocks of pandemic are not sufficient to galvanise a political commitment to reform, where will the impetus to change come from? Chapter 4 set out how a succession of initiatives, White Papers, Green Papers and consultations of one kind and another have failed to produce improvements on the scale needed. If anything, they may have made matters worse by propping up a failing system, postponing its demise instead of replacing it. It may be that the crisis in social care, in the words of Antonio Gramsci, 'consists precisely in the fact that the old is dying and the new cannot be born; in this interregnum a great variety of morbid symptoms appear' (Gramsci, 1971).

Social care has been let down badly by politics and the policy process. It exemplifies the failure of democratic politics in the UK to deal with this and other pressing problems facing the country. In making the case for a different way of doing politics, Polly Mackenzie, then head of the Demos think tank, tells the story of Gloria Foster. An 81-year-old widow, Gloria died in 2013, after an immigration raid shut down the care agency whose carers helped her out of bed in the morning. She was left alone and unable to summon help for nine days. By the time she was found, soaked in urine, it was too late to save her. It illustrates the disconnection between the intentions of citizens and the consequences of policy decisions:

> Gloria Foster suffered alone because of profound political dysfunction. Voters would never support a system, in aggregate, that left someone to experience such agony. And yet voters have opposed tax rises, supported robust immigration enforcement, and supported governments that cut back local government budgets to breaking point. The mismatch arises because – with the best of intentions – we have allowed citizens to outsource all complexity and decision-making to elected officials, about whom they then complain. (Mackenzie, 2021)

With the spotlight now on the latest in a long line of White Papers, there is a very real danger more of the same – 'one more heave' that will simply repeat the cycle of failure instead of breaking out of it. In some quarters, there is a continuing assumption that more hard, data-driven evidence of the value of social care is needed to thaw the cold hearts of HM Treasury. The problem is seen as an information deficit. Evidence from other campaigns for social change suggests that reformers should instead focus their efforts on the 'salience deficit' where policy-makers take a different view of the problem or do not see it as important, and the 'power deficit' where those wanting change have little power or influence over policy-makers (Laybourn-Langton et al, 2021). Chapter 4 argued that too much time has been spent considering policy content – the 'what' of social care reform – and too little time on policy process – the 'how'. Attention therefore should surely now refocus on the politics and process of reform: how to secure political traction and public support for a clear plan for social care, one that can be sustained through design of a better system, decision-making and implementation.

Doing policy-making differently

Drawing on the lessons from the past and from the experience of other countries described in previous chapters, what could a more successful approach involve? There are four aspects to the politics and process of reform that need to be fundamentally different.

1: Clarity of purpose

One of the main reasons why previous attempts to reform social care have floundered (explained in Chapter 4) is that they have tended to focus on a very limited set of issues. These have usually been how social care should be paid for and where the money should come from. Little regard has been paid to the kind of care and support that people want and need. It is true, of course, that most governments have come up with a vision or statement of purpose. The examples recounted in Chapter 2 include the Seebohm idea of universal, community-based social services departments in the 1970s; the needs-led community care reforms in the 1990s; the cross-government 'Putting People First' vision for personalised support in 2007; and most recently the 2014 Care Act, with its noble aim of replacing the narrow assessment of eligibility with the promotion of wellbeing as the driving principal of social care. As discussed in Chapter 2, however, these great visions consisted of laudable but grandiose aspirations that quickly became disconnected from the financial and policy levers needed to make them happen, if they were ever connected in the first place. All failed to gain traction in the face of economic or political crises and sometimes both. They failed at the stage of implementation.

In all the years recounted here, there has never been a single comprehensive strategy that identifies the full range of problems and challenges that afflict social care and sets out a plan to deal with them, a plan that is backed with sufficient money and the policy levers to make sure it is put into practice. As noted in Chapter 3, it has never been entirely clear what, if the reform of social care is the answer, the question is. There are different takes on this, as former King's Fund colleague Simon Bottery points out (Figure 7.1). Most of the reform initiatives have tried to answer some of the questions, but none has addressed all of them. The most glaring omission has been around the workforce. While the policy debates have fixated on funding, especially the issue of protecting inheritances, the neglect of workforce issues has meant mounting staffing pressures and the subsequent exposure of workers to intolerable conditions under COVID-19. Many people are now struggling to get care, not necessarily because there is not enough money to pay for it, but because there are not enough people to do it.

Too often, reform objectives have been unimaginative and small scale, assuming, for example, that the social care market is a given that can be tweaked or 'fixed' to make it work. Rarely has there been a systematic reimagining of what good care should look like and how it can be secured. Are there better and very different ways of meeting needs? The Archbishops of Canterbury and York have set up a commission (of which I am a member) for that very purpose (Archbishop of Canterbury, 2021). Chapter 3 described how the #SocialCareFuture movement has drawn heavily on the lived experience of people with care and support needs to frame the purpose of

Figure 7.1: What's your problem, social care? Eight key areas for reform

1. Means testing: it's not like the NHS:

   People receive health care free at the point of use but are expected to make a substantial personal contribution towards their social care. This is widely regarded as unfair. Disabled people complain that care charges eat into their weekly income and take no account of the extra costs of disability.

2. Catastrophic costs: selling homes to pay for care

   One in seven of us will need care costing at least £100,000 and some will need to sell their main asset – their home – to pay for it.

3. Unmet need: people going without the care and support they need

   Fewer people are getting publicly funded care even though there are more older and disabled people with care needs. Age UK estimate that around 1.4 million older people are not getting the support they need.

4. Quality of care: 15-minute care visits and neglect

   Financial and workforce shortfalls affect the quality of care, ranging from the risk of poor care in under-staffed services to rushed visits from home care workers and little choice or control over the help people get.

5. Workforce pay and conditions: underpaid, overworked staff

   There are at least 106,000 vacancies, pay and conditions of service and training available does not reflect the skills required.

6. Market fragility: care companies going out of business

   More organisations providing care are going out of business or handing back contracts to councils because they cannot cover their costs or recruit enough staff.

7. Disjointed care: delayed transfers of care and lack of integration with health

   More people have a mixture of physical and mental health needs that can only be met by different parts of the NHS and social care working well together so that people get timely coordinated care instead of fragmented care.

8. The postcode lottery: unwarranted variation in access and performance

   Despite national eligibility rules, the care and support people are offered often depends on where they live rather than what they need. Each council decides their own budget and decides their own priorities. Some councils can raise more money than others.

Source: Bottery (2019)

social care in a way that could not be more different from the current model. A clear and settled view about what we want from a better system of social care – the purpose of reform – can be condensed under three broad groups of questions set out in Chapter 4 about purpose and entitlement, organisation and delivery and, finally, funding.

A theme throughout this book is that people have a diverse range of needs, depending on their individually unique and highly personalised circumstances. Different people want different things from social care, so the answers to those three groups of questions may not necessarily be the same. There was a lively debate in the 2000s, for example, about whether the needs of older people were so very different from working age people that there should be two different systems. There are also conflicting ideas and opinions among political parties, and sometimes within them, clashes that have set back progress at key points, as documented in Chapter 4. This begs a critically important question about how much agreement can be reached about all these questions and how much difference can be tolerated.

It is also important not to exaggerate the extent to which political parties are divided. In fact, as noted earlier, there has been a cross-party consensus about social care policy for most of the time since 1948. Chapter 2 described how most of the big organisational and legislative changes since 1948 enjoyed cross-party support. Indeed, policy group-think might be just as problematic as political pugilism. There are many examples in the last few years where cross-party parliamentary groups and committees have had little difficulty in reaching common cause about social care. It is usually only at election time, when parties are touting ideas for how care should be paid for, that conflict erupts. The obvious implication, as Chapter 4 noted, is that a general election campaign is a terrible time to float contentious proposals, especially when their subject matter is poorly understood by the electorate, and political parties are busy promoting their policy differences and have no interest whatsoever in finding common ground. Better ways of securing political support, if not consensus, for change must be found.

2: Agreeing the basics – design principles for better care

Another way in which the process of reform needs to be different is to start with the points on which most people agree, not with the controversial questions that invariably revolve around funding and taxes. Many organisations have developed a set of principles that should guide the design of better social care. These include charities, think tanks, parliamentary committees, reviews and commissions, such as the #SocialCareFuture vision and the 'Distinctive, Valued, Personal' road map produced by Directors of Adult Social Care (ADASS, 2015). A wide range of bodies involved in social care have signed up to 'Seven Principles of Social Care Reform' (Local Government Association, 2020). There are some differences in language and emphasis of these various statements, but there is considerable overlap and similarity between them. Condensed here into a single set of principles in Figure 7.2, these could form the foundation of a policy-making process that begins at the beginning, with a much clearer understanding of the purpose of social care and the range of issues that need to be addressed. They offer a platform for discussion and debate, a template for a different set of conversations with and between politicians and with the wider public. How to translate these principles into a set of comprehensive proposals for change also demands a very different style of policy-making.

3: Co-produced policy-making

The traditional process used by governments to reform social care, discussed in Chapter 4, has usually been top-down. It involves publishing a Green Paper that sets out the issues and the options for dealing with them. There is usually a standard 12-week period of public consultation (though it can be longer), after which the government publishes a White Paper setting out what it proposes to do. Sometimes, the report of an independent review or commission is part of the mix to which the government responds. It will then seek to pass new legislation through Parliament, unless the proposals can be made within existing laws or regulations. As an approach to policy-making and

Figure 7.2: Principles for reform of social care

Good social care:

1. Promotes independence, enabling people to live the best lives they can, in their own homes and communities for as long as possible; and, by building on the assets of communities and families, prevents or postpones the need for long-term care;

2. Addresses the needs of people of all ages, of working age as well as of older; with the individual in the driving seat in shaping the care and support they need;

3. Is founded on the human rights, needs and wishes of the individual, and their families and carers, upholding the principles of the Care Act, Equalities Act and Mental Capacity Act; and avoids discrimination on the basis of clinical diagnosis by offering equal treatment of equal needs;

4. Recognises the role of carers and the scale of their current contribution to the care of older and disabled people; and gives higher priority to the needs of the paid workforce to be valued through reward, recognition and investment in their skills and development;

5. Is as simple as possible for people to understand, access and navigate;

6. Offers certainty about what people can expect in terms of care, support and safeguards and what they are responsible for by way of provision and payment;

7. Works well with other public services – especially the NHS and housing and benefit systems – so that people receive coordinated, joined-up care;

8. Has adequate funding that enables councils to fulfil their legal responsibilities, and providers to cover the costs of care and meet the standards set by regulators; and is sufficient to meet the needs of individuals, either through direct payments or care arranged by councils;

9. Seeks a fair balance in how the costs of good care are shared between individuals, families and the state, and between generations; a balance that can be recalibrated over time to reflect changing patterns of income and wealth.

implementation, it may be successful in getting new legislation on the statute book, but it has not been sufficient to drive through real change in the lives of people with care and support needs. It is a very linear process, driven by a set of organisational and procedural requirements that expect people to respond in very formal ways. Usually, this takes the form of written submissions and thus favours formal organisations with the resources and skills for this. It is sometimes marked by internal tensions, between ministers and civil servants or between the government department and lobbyists, charities, campaigning groups and professional stakeholders. It is focused on the machinery of government in Whitehall and Westminster, with little traction in the many thousands of places and homes throughout the country where people experience care and support. In the age of 24/7 news coverage and the widespread use of social media and digital technology, it is an analogue process in a digital age. As such, it is entirely possible that most of the official documents and reports about social care over the last 25 years have passed unnoticed by most people, even many of those who experience and work in social care. Unless accompanied by a major public information campaign, that is likely to be the case for most of the general public too. Certainly none have been bestselling publications to compare with the Beveridge Report when print was the ubiquitous medium. There is no reason to believe that this cycle of failure stands any better chance of success in the future. A policy-making process that fails to engage people who use social care and the wider public can surely only repeat past mistakes instead of learning from them?

There have been some attempts to break away from the tramlines of traditional policy-making and formal consultation. In 2009, the Labour government launched the 'Big Care Debate', described as the largest ever public consultation on social care. Over a period of five months, it tried to take the debate to the people in town centres, shopping centres and county shows, through supplementary research and questionnaires, and 68,000 people had their say (HM Government 2009). The questions the public were asked, however, were framed by proposals in the already-published Green Paper 'Shaping the Future of Care Today'.

The Care Act 2014 is another example of a different approach to policy-making. This was widely hailed as a successful example of co-production, with central and local government working together, not just in designing the policy content of the legislation but in collaborating to support its implementation. On its own, however, co-production was not enough to fulfil the ambition of the Act, namely, to shift the system towards prevention and wellbeing.[1] The team that evaluated the implementation support programme noted 'the difficulties that arise when a policy that is collaboratively designed, popular with the receiving audience and supported by an implementation programme, is not properly funded to achieve its objectives' (Peckham et al 2019). This was yet another reminder that, while reform is not just about money, the lack of it limits what can be done.

The experience of both the Care Act and Big Care Debate offered a glimpse of how policy-making could be improved, but bigger changes are needed: an entirely different set of reform processes; ones that are capable of generating proposals that can command a broad base of support and legitimacy and so are much more likely to be implemented effectively in a way that makes a real difference to people's lives. A different approach to policy-making could involve three prongs:

1. Make greater use of mechanisms to build cross-party cooperation and support, ensuring ideas and proposals are built on principles that are widely shared, such that they will not be torpedoed by political arguments about tax, death and inheritances.
2. Apply the principles of co-production to develop and test ideas with people with lived experience, and everyone with a stake in social care, including councils, care providers and voluntary and community organisations who provide advice and support.
3. Develop systemic programmes of engagement with the wider public using the principles of participatory democracy, using methods such as citizens assemblies, deliberative events and focus groups.

There are some encouraging examples of small-scale initiatives that demonstrate the potential of a co-produced, citizen-led and bottom-up strategy for policy reform. In 2018, a Citizens' Assembly on Social Care brought together a representative group of 47 randomly selected English citizens over two weekends to consider the question of how adult social care in England should be funded. It was the first of its kind to be commissioned by the UK Parliament, set up by two parliamentary committees as part of their joint inquiry into long-term funding. Assembly members took part in approximately 28 hours of deliberation, equating to a total of 1,316 'people hours' of learning, deliberation and decision-making. (Involve and House of Commons, 2018). Members considered a wide range of evidence, opinions and perspectives. This kind of exercise is described as 'deliberative' because multiple views are considered and members are encouraged to express, develop and re-examine their views in the light of what they have heard. They are asked also to consider any trade-offs between different options. Their final recommendations are the product of informed citizens working together. Evaluation of the Citizens' Assembly showed that it had helped the joint committees to reach agreement on their recommendations (bearing in mind that its membership was drawn from all political parties). As some interviewees from members and staff of the two committees put it:

> 'Getting people who are not in their day-to-day lives, much engaged in politics to understand that decisions are more difficult than they look and think a bit about the costs and benefits of choices that you make, you can't have everything' (Interviewee 1), because 'in order to reform social care, it needs to be accompanied by that process of learning and engaging people' (Interviewee 3). (Elstub and Carrick, 2019)

The joint committee went on to recommend that, building on the experience of the Citizens' Assembly, the government should conduct a public engagement programme to raise awareness of, and support for, change. Further, that a parliamentary commission (an ad hoc committee of from both Houses of Parliament) should be established to help form cross-party agreement about reform, emulating the success of the Turner Commission in achieving a consensus on pensions (House of Commons, 2018).

Whether another commission is needed is a moot point. Chapter 4 set out the procession of inquiries, commissions and reviews since the royal commission in 1999. As Harold Wilson famously observed of royal commissions, 'they take minutes and waste years', but there is considerable support from MPs of all political hues for a parliamentary commission, a vehicle that is more fleet-of-foot and with a better track record in other areas of public policy (House of Commons, 2018). In Germany, the construction of a 'grand coalition' of political parties and policy-makers was instrumental in developing proposals and negotiating the eventual shape of reforms with employers and other stakeholders (Theobald and Hampel, 2013). In Japan, there were extensive discussions and engagement with stakeholders and the public long before legislation was passed in 1997 and a new system of long term care implemented from 2000 (Ikegami, 2007). Coupling a substantial programme of public engagement, run on deliberative principles, with a mechanism for cross-party support, both beginning with a blank sheet of paper, could be a game changer.

Other examples support the value of deliberative events that can help shift the dial of public perceptions. For example the deliberative workshops run by Ipsos Mori described in Chapter 3. I contributed to the Leeds events as an expert advisor and I was struck by the open-minded and thoughtful way in which people from a very wide range of backgrounds deliberated on the issues. It showed that, when people are given clear information about social care, they recognise the problems in the current system, support the need to do something about it and see the benefits of doing it.

Another example of involving people in developing policies from the bottom up is the work of Engage Britain, a charity that brings people together to find solutions to some of the big challenges facing the country. In early 2021, they convened a series of 'community conversations' bringing together about 700 people from around the country to share ideas and experiences about health and social care. They included people who work in health and social care as well as the general public. A People's Panel' of around 100 was set up to consider what came out of the community conversations and work out what the most important issues were. The prioritised issues were then taken into a co-design phase where Engage Britain brought together more people – including frontline staff, patients, people who draw on care support and those who decide how services are run – to co-create deliverable, costed plans for change. Those solutions will be tested to make sure that they will make a difference to people and are politically sustainable; the ultimate goal for these plans being to get them put into practice by government so everyone benefits.[2]

A fresh approach to the reform process along these lines has three compelling benefits that stand a much higher chance of success than traditional methods:

- It can produce better-quality policy proposals through open-minded discussion of the issues with people who know about and understand social care, especially those with lived experience of it.
- It can help to build public support for proposals and demonstrate to politicians that voters can be won over. If the support of other stakeholders, such as the business community or trade unions can be secured, that in turn can help to win over the wider public and provide political cover for the government to implement potentially controversial policies.
- It will help to raise general awareness of what social care is, its importance and value. This is crucial because, time and time again, widespread confusion and poor understanding of social care has seriously weakened efforts to get politicians to take social care seriously. If the public do not understand the importance and relevance of social care to their own lives, they have little reason to support solutions to its problems. (Davies et al, 2018). As Norman Lamb observed, it was easy for the Cameron government to ditch the Dilnot reforms in 2015 because few people understood what they were or why they were important.

It is not just social care reform that has been failed by politics. In *The Blunders of our Governments*, political scientists Antony King and Ivor Crewe offer a forensic assessment of the mistakes made by governments over three decades, over a wide range of policy issues, from the poll tax to the Millennium Dome. Behind many of these failures, they argue, lies a 'deficit of deliberation', of carefully weighing up options and reaching out to those with greater knowledge and experience than that of ministers and civil servants in Whitehall. The advantages of a deliberative approach to making policy are clear:

> On the one hand, ministers know there are long term issues that they ought to be tackling. On the other hand, they know that tackling them effectively may damage them electorally. As a possible way out of this conundrum, the practice of deliberation, of weighing up, proceeding without haste and taking counsel together, may be of use ... If a broad range of stakeholders, including the opposition parties, can agree a way forward – if their fingerprints are clearly visible on whatever agreement is ultimately negotiated –then it may be possible to take the issue out of politics, or if not out politics altogether, then at least out of electoral politics. Agreement reached by way of deliberation also stand a good chance of being widely accepted, not least because more individuals and organisations will have had their opinions and interests taken into account ... In addition, policies that secure widespread agreement are more likely to 'stick', not to be abandoned or reversed when there is next a change of government. (King and Crewe, 2013)

The relationship between public understanding of social care and how far politicians are committed to do something about it is crucial. In the 1990s, American political analyst Joseph Overton explored how different policy ideas would be considered by politicians to be more acceptable than others, a concept that came to be known as the Overton window (Figure 7.3). The creation of an NHS-style health care in the USA, for example, would sit completely outside the window, but the less radical, though highly contentious, alternative of the Obamacare reforms was brought within it. In the UK, the prohibition of smoking in public places at one time would have been considered unthinkable, yet changing social attitudes to smoking was to bring it inside the window. Overton argued that the goal of reformers should not be to lobby politicians to support policies

Figure 7.3: The Overton window

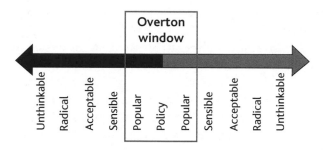

Source: Waytowich (2019)

outside the window, but to convince voters that policies outside the window should be in it (Astor, 2019).

Social care has dropped in and out of the Overton window several times in the last 30 years (chronicled in Chapter 4), and particular policy solutions have fallen in and out of favour. It is worth noting that, for many years, the policy of free personal care was seen as beyond the pale. It was not even included as an option for consultation when Labour was developing its ideas for a national care service in 2009 on the grounds that it placed 'a heavy burden on people of working age' (HM Government, 2009a). At the time, the dominant idea sitting squarely in the centre of the Overton window was a partnership model of funding that shared the costs of care between individuals and the state. More recently, there has been a sharp resurgence of support for free personal care. This makes the system more straightforward to understand and tackles the anomaly that social care is not free at the point of need, unlike the NHS. It now enjoys a wide range of support from bodies that include the independent Barker Commission, the Institute of Public Policy Research, the House of Lords Economic Affairs Committee, Policy Exchange and two parliamentary select committees. The point here is not the merits or otherwise of free personal care, but that the policy options that are regarded as politically acceptable can and do change. There is a fickleness in the political appetite for particular options, especially funding, that in part reflects changing perceptions of what the problem is that need fixing. The overarching challenge of our time is how to keep social care as a priority for reform within the Overton window long enough for a range of ideas to be considered, conclusions reached and changes implemented effectively.

Participative and deliberative methods discussed earlier represent one way to help achieve this, but social movements that harness grassroots support for change, large and small, have the potential to place rocket-boosters under these initiatives and expand public support even further. One of the most popular and successful changes in social care discussed in Chapter 2 was the introduction of direct payments that gave people much more control over their lives. This innovation emanated not from a great mind in Westminster but from the actions of a small group of disabled people in Hampshire and was to trigger the emergence of the independent living movement in the UK (Evans, 2003). In Australia, the Every Australian Counts movement was to achieve success on a much bigger scale. Hundreds of thousands of people with disabilities and their families, carers, and those who work to support them, all came together and successfully campaigned for better support. The result was the National Disability Insurance scheme (described, in Chapter 5), implemented from 2013.

It is important to recognise that the impetus behind both of these examples was not to get better traditional care services per se, but rather to get the support that would enable people to live as they chose, through employment, education, access to leisure, transportation and other rights. Since 2011, the Caring Across Generations movement has been campaigning for better care at home for older and disabled Americans. A broad coalition involving care providers and labour unions, as well as individuals themselves, it has argued successfully for care services to be considered part of the country's infrastructure. Polling suggests that the majority of voters support 'bold investments in home and community services' and agree that this will promote economic growth (Caring Across Generations, 2021). This was reflected in President Biden's proposals for $400 billion new investment in home care as part of his even bigger infrastructure plan (Cohn, 2021; Stein, 2021). In considering the potential of a similar movement for change in England, there are two aspects of Caring Across Generations and Every Australian Counts that stand out. The first is that they bring together a wide range of groups and organisations, including care providers and business organisations, alongside people with care and support needs. The second is that their pitch is aimed not at improving a narrow range of traditional services but how to offer people a better, meaningful life in the context of wider social and economic objectives. In England the #SocialCareFuture campaign is trying to build a similar movement for change – a 'coalition of the willing' – but whether it can gain sufficient support from mainstream care providers remains to be seen.

4: Cathedral thinking

The final element of a different approach to policy-making is to abandon the short-termism that has acted as a screeching brake on efforts to reform of social care. A theme throughout this book is that the nature of social care in England today is the product of over 70 years of history and the accretion of ad hoc policy decisions, sometimes completely unrelated to social care. Untangling these messy threads of policy, finance and organisation and designing a better system cannot be achieved overnight. An indisputable lesson from the history of social care, as presently understood, is that enduring change and improvement takes many years, if not decades to achieve.

Chapter 4 set out the multiple policy initiatives and series of ad hoc funding announcements, often last-minute and time-limited, that have offered only sticking-plaster responses to deeper maladies that require much more radical treatment. Yet, despite the way COVID-19 has brutally exposed the consequences of long-term neglect, policy-makers remain fixated on the short term. On just one day in November 2021, there was a blizzard of five separate policy announcements. They included £120 million of new funding to increase staff capacity, to be paid to councils from February and to be spent within five months; a separate recruitment and retention fund of £162 million, also one-off, also to be spent within five months; and, with winter almost upon us, a 'winter plan' for adult social care (DHSC, 2021b). Never mind the continuing absence of a long-term workforce strategy to tackle the escalating shortage of staff discussed earlier.

The importance of time as a currency of change has been showed over and over again in efforts to improve the way social care and the NHS work together. 'Hyperactive' policy-making, in which new policies are layered on top of old policies and new pilots rapidly eclipse older ones without sufficient time to work, has undermined the long-term commitment that is needed to achieve joined-up care (Miller et al, 2021). The Better Care Fund (discussed in Chapter 3), is a specific example of an initiative that expected too much, too soon, with too little (NAO, 2017).

This is the political equivalent of attention deficit disorder. It creates the impression of action, bringing to mind the politician's syllogism familiar to viewers of the BBC politics sitcom *Yes Prime Minister*, yet leaving unaddressed the underlying causes:

> Something must be done.
> This is something.
> This must be done.

A more insidious consequence of short-termism is the way it stymies any hope of achieving an ambitious vision for better social care. Nowhere is this more evident than in the straitjacket of the one-year financial settlement. This means that, even in the better years when there is some budget growth, as there has been since 2017, councils tend to plan with the 2 or 3 per cent extra. When spending power is falling, the planning is with the 5 per cent, or whatever amount that has to be cut from existing budgets. So, the planning is necessarily incremental, with the 3 per cent or 5 per cent change, instead of bigger changes that would be possible by planning with the 103 per cent or 97 per cent. Former Treasury permanent secretary Nick Macpherson calls this 'the tyranny of the baseline' (Institute of Fiscal Studies, 2021). Everything is reduced to what can be done in just one year. This makes it next to impossible to invest in, for example, preventive support that could save money – but not until a few years down the line, or to fund the up-front costs of developing better, more cost-effective alternatives to residential care while funding existing services until the benefits come through.

Even less attention is given to how the money is spent, and what is achieved with it. As the National Audit Office has pointed out, the lack of a long-term vision for care and only short-term funding has hampered councils' abilities to innovate and plan for the long term, and constrained investment both in accommodation for older people and much-needed workforce development (NAO, 2021). Crucially, short-termism means that, even when the government does put more money into social care, it is used to buttress a failing system instead of building a bridge to a better one.

The inability to look beyond the next few years is not just a problem in social care policy. Most governments tend to overestimate what can be achieved in the short term and underestimate what can be done in the longer term. The UK is not the only country that has thus been left ill-equipped to deal with anthropogenic (man-made) threats such as climate change, pandemics, financial crashes and the consequences of underinvestment in housing, public health and the needs of ageing societies. Political anxieties for quick fixes trump the harder and longer work of finding sustainable solutions. Across the world there is growing interest in how public policies should take account of the needs of future generations instead of reacting to immediate issues of the moment.

Philosopher Roman Krznaric poses the question of how we will be judged by those who come after us. Will the legacy of our generation be a benefit to them or a burden? He cites the example of medical researcher Jonas Salk, who led the development of the polio vaccine in the 1950s that has since saved millions of lives. Salk never sought to have the vaccine patented, instead preferring to leave a good legacy for future generations. Later on, he described his philosophy of life as one question, 'Are we being good ancestors?' (Krznaric, 2020). We are grateful for the positive bequests from our predecessors – the vision of universal care and education, the many advances in science, medicine and technology that has given us more comfortable lives that are much less nasty, brutish and short (although an NHS that focuses mostly on treating acute illness is becoming increasingly ill-suited to an era of pandemics, widespread chronic illness and health inequalities). We think less well of the negatives – the bitter legacies of slavery, of religious and racial discrimination, environmental destruction, deepening social divisions and economic inequalities.

Krznaric argues that, whereas the struggles of previous centuries were fought with guns, money and trade, in the 21st century, the struggle is between the forces of short-termism that threaten to drag us down and the drivers for longer-term horizons that help us to take responsibility for the future. He describes this as the tug of war for time (Figure 7.4).

Many countries have introduced new ways of putting long-term thinking at the forefront of decision-making. Since 1993, Finland has had a Committee of the Future as a standing committee of Parliament; Hungary and Israel each has a Commissioner for Future Generations; Singapore's Centre for Strategic Futures has developed methodologies for thinking about future risks, trends and opportunities; Scotland's Future Forum aims to look beyond immediate horizons to future challenges and opportunities; and Wales passed the Well-being of Future Generations Act in 2015, creating a Future Generations Commissioner. These examples differ in their structure, function and powers, but can include advocacy, campaigning and commissioning for 'futures' research; requiring public bodies to demonstrate the impact of their policies on future generations; and monitoring or even vetoing legislation. A common thread is helping policy-makers to pay more attention to *fireproofing* decisions for the future and spend less time *firefighting* those of the present and the past. Despite some evidence that their effectiveness can be limited by the capriciousness of short-term electoral cycles, they have had a positive impact (Jones et al, 2018).

The timeline over which policies have an impact is much shorter for social care than for other existential crises, like climate change or antimicrobial resistance. This is all the more reason to think about the longer-term impact of reforms. It begs the question of what legacy do we want to leave for future generations as a result of the decisions made about social care now? How can we be 'good ancestors' when it comes to care and support? Krznaric describes this is a 'legacy mindset', basing policy thinking not just on the exigencies of the immediate moment but the implications for future generations. If someone were writing a book about social care in say 50 or 100 years'

Figure 7.4: The tug of war for time

Graphic: Nigel Hawtin

Six drivers of short-termism		Six ways to think long

Tyranny of the clock
the acceleration of time
since the Middle Ages

Deep-time humility
grasp we are an eyeblink
in cosmic time

Digital distraction
the hijacking of attention
by technology

Legacy mindset
be remembered
well by posterity

Political presentism
myopic focus
on the next election

Intergenerational justice
consider the seventh
generation ahead

Speculative capitalism
volatile boom-bust
financial markets

Cathedral thinking
plan projects beyond
a human lifetime

Networked uncertainty
the rise of global risk
and contagion

Holistic forecasting
envision multiple pathways
for civilisation

Perpetual progress
the pursuit of
endless economic growth

Transcendent goal
strive for
one-planet thriving

Source: Krznaric (2020)

time, what would be its verdict? What will our successors, 'the universal strangers of the future', experience in seeking help with their care and support needs? The question of how we wish to be remembered scarcely features in discussions about social care reform. Much of the debate has been focused on *intra-*generational justice. It asks how care should be funded so that it is fair to today's cohorts of older and retired people, as well as to younger, working-age people who pay the bulk of taxation yet are often less wealthy than those whose care they are helping to pay for. This is a typically myopic way of viewing the issue, for reasons that will be discussed in the final chapter. The debate rarely looks through the longer-term lens of justice between generations over time. This was encapsulated by Swedish climate activist Greta Thunberg in her speech to the United Nations Climate Change conference (COP 24):

> The year 2078, I will celebrate my 75th birthday. If I have children, then maybe they will spend that day with me. Maybe they will ask about you. Maybe they will ask why you didn't do anything while there was still time to act. You say you love your children above all else, and yet you are stealing their future in front of their very eyes. (Rigitano, 2018)

What this means for social care is best understood by reflecting on the miserable legacy of our ancestors. Beyond the policy failures of the last 30-odd years, the roots of what today we call social care go back not just to the National Assistance Act in 1948, but the Victorian and even the Elizabethan Poor Laws. Shrouded in the mists of history, these archaic policy artefacts have left a profound imprint on the nature of social care hundreds of years later (as recounted in Chapter 2). In the last century, Beveridge and Bevan lacked the foresight to anticipate the social and medical transformations that were to make social care such a critical issue for many countries across the world.

Today's generation of social care reformers need to do so much better, so that future generations will see a very different and much better social care system; one that elicits the same degree of pride and gratitude as today's generation feel towards the architects of the NHS over 70 years ago. That surely should be a central purpose of reform now. In an era of hyperactive policy-making, it may be too much to urge the adoption of what many in indigenous nations call the 'seventh generation principle'. This obliges policy-makers and legislators to take on a stewardship role by considering the impact of the decisions they make today on the welfare and wellbeing of the seventh generation down the line.

The idea of building policies and a good infrastructure of care and support as a long-term endeavour is reflected in the notion of 'cathedral thinking'. As the name suggests, it draws on many examples from architecture and is lyrically articulated by astrophysicist Martin Rees in his 2011 Templeton Prize acceptance speech:

> No one can fail to be uplifted by great cathedrals – such as that at Ely, near my home in Cambridge. Ely Cathedral overwhelms us today. But think of its impact 900 years ago – think of the vast enterprise its construction entailed. Most of its builders had never travelled more than 50 miles; the Fens were their world. Even the most educated knew of essentially nothing beyond Europe. They thought the world was a few thousand years old – and that it might not last another thousand. But despite these constricted horizons, in both time and space – despite the deprivation and harshness of their lives – despite their primitive technology and meagre resources – they built this huge and glorious building – pushing the boundaries of what was possible. Those who conceived it knew they wouldn't live to see it finished. Their legacy still elevates our spirits, nearly a millennium later. (Rees, 2011)

Cathedral thinking is not just about cathedrals. Krznaric cites the construction of the London sewers in the 1850s that took 18 years and are still in use, the creation of the NHS and the global eradication of smallpox. This shows that there is a human capacity for thinking beyond the immediate needs of today's generation. Policy-making around big decisions do not have to be in thrall to the timing of the next election. As the supply of quick fixes available for social care are depleting rapidly, there has never been a better time to adopt a long-term mindset as a driving process to achieve the major changes that are required.

A new road to reform

The central thrust of this chapter is that the solutions to the many problems with England's social care arrangements will not be found in conventional top-down policy-making. Neither will solutions be found in yet more reviews, commissions, policy papers or analyses of funding options. There is no intellectual cavalry coming over the hill with some startling new idea or magic bullet innovation. Whatever the problems in social care are, a dearth of policy documents and ideas is not one of them. There is no sign of a messianic figure like Beveridge, brandishing a blueprint that will carry all before it. Repeating yet again the tired cycle of failure of the past invokes the ubiquitous Einstein definition of stupidity. Instead, a fundamentally different approach is needed to the politics and processes of change. A better road to reform must be found that will not end up in a political cul-de-sac or the infamous long grass after a change of government or some other squall in the political or economic weather. It has four interlinked dimensions:

- Defining clearly the purpose of social care in a 21st-century economy and society, and setting out the full range of problems and challenges that need to be addressed. These include individual entitlements, how care is organised and delivered and how it is paid for and by whom.
- Reaching agreement about the key design principles needed to guide the planning of a better social care system, building on the consensus and partnerships that already exist across organisations involved in social care, people with lived experience and policy-makers.
- Replacing tired formal consultation processes with a bottom-up, citizen-led and co-produced approach to policy-making, nurturing cross-party support and cooperation; drawing on the knowledge, ideas and experience of people who use social care, their families, carers, health and social care professionals, commissioners and providers; and using participatory democracy and the power of social movements to nurture public support for change.
- Adopting a temporal shift from short-term fixes to long-term thinking, recognising that serious reforms will not be achieved through immediate changes alone; applying a legacy mindset and cathedral thinking to develop a staged, long-term plan

that will enable us to become 'good ancestors' to the next generation and beyond.

A radically different approach to policy-making along these lines, aligned with a new financial settlement and the right policy framework, offers a new and more promising road to reform. What kind of social care system might emerge from going down this road? What would better social care look like? The potential building blocks of a new model of social care – the raw material for the new processes set out here – are the subject of the next and final chapter.

8

A new future for social care

What you leave behind is not what is engraved in stone monuments but what is woven into the hearts of others.

Pericles

Does the cap fit?

In the early months of 2022, the prospects for better social care seemed as distant as ever. A last-minute amendment to the Health and Social Care Bill before Parliament meant that the proposed cap on individual care costs would turn out to offer less protection than the original proposals to people with modest savings and wealth, especially in places with lower house prices. Those in the North East, Yorkshire and the Humber, and the Midlands will be worst hit, having to contribute more towards care charges than those in London and the South East (Sturrock and Tallack, 2022). This appears to fly in the face of the government's plans to 'level-up' parts of the country that have lagged behind economically. Once again, a government's attempts to tackle social care caused political fur to fly, with a backbench rebellion over the proposed hike in National Insurance and the accusations that the health and social care levy amounted to a new 'dementia tax' on the working class. The government went on to win the House of Commons vote but lost the argument in the eyes of most independent commentators. 'Poorly conceived' and 'a step in the wrong direction', was the Health Foundation's verdict (Health Foundation, 2021). The less-well-off losers from the change may well wonder, as the King's Fund put it, 'why the Prime Minister's promise that no one need sell their house to pay for care will benefit wealthier people but doesn't seem to apply to them' (King's Fund 2021a). For the Nuffield Trust, Natasha Curry lamented that the long hoped-for comprehensive plan to deliver lasting change still appeared to be a long way off (Nuffield Trust, 2021).

In the government's defence, its proposals for funding reform in the Health and Social Care Bill do represent an overall improvement over the current system, particularly the substantial increase in the means-test threshold, though that is a very low bar given the well-chronicled and widespread deficiencies of the existing system. The plans also offer a nudge towards universalism by eventually bringing more self-funders into the public system. The government has taken a politically courageous decision to raise taxation to pay for it. At the time of writing, however, the amended version before Parliament is far less generous than the 2015 plans, especially for working-age people with care needs who, under the 2015 proposals, would have enjoyed a cap set at zero: they would have paid no charges for their care. The chosen method of paying for the reforms – a hypothecated National Insurance rise – has also been criticised for being regressive (National Insurance contributions are paid only by working-age people, and the marginal rate of NI is lower for higher earners) and for making funding even more complex (Institute of Fiscal Studies, 2021a).

The political debate, in the mother of parliaments at least, has not moved on. It remains trapped in the same politically constricted trope as it was in 1997 when Tony Blair raised the spectre of older people having to sell their homes to pay for care. The narrative seems permanently stuck on asset protection as the main problem to be fixed.

Many hoped that might change when the government finally published its promised White Paper 'People at the Heart of Care' a few weeks later, with a welcome recognition that there were other problems that need to be addressed. It set out 'an ambitious 10-year vision for how we will transform support and care in England' (DHSC, 2021c) based on three objectives to ensure that:

1. People have choice, control, and support to live independent lives.
2. People can access outstanding quality and tailored care and support.
3. People find adult social care fair and accessible.

These aims are unexceptional in that they echo the personalisation and independence-promoting themes of the many past White Papers and policy documents described in Chapter 2. It is less clear how they will be connected to the levers of policy and money to make change happen.

The bulk of the £5.2 billion the government has identified for social care over the next three years will be gobbled up by the costs of the cap on care costs and reducing how much self-funders pay for their residential care (the 'fair cost of care' programme). That leaves just £1.7 billion, divvied up into smaller pots of money for supported housing (£300 million), technology (£150 million), innovative models of care (£30 million) and support for unpaid carers (£25 million). The largest £500 million is for workforce developments (referred to in Chapter 6). These amounts, though welcomed, are derisory in relation to the scale of what needs to be done. They fall well short of the £1.5 billion a year needed simply to meet existing cost and demand pressures, never mind make improvements (Local Government Association, 2021a). Even the Secretary of State's introduction discourages high expectations, cautioning that the White Paper 'will not solve all of the problems' but takes 'the next steps on our social care reform journey.'

Outside the Westminster bubble, our health and social care system is melting. Waiting times for hospital care and social care assessments are at record levels. There are stories of very old people who have had a fall left lying on floors for hours because the ambulance they need is stuck outside local hospital emergency departments. They cannot transfer their patients into the hospital because all beds are full. As winter 2021 approached, many NHS leaders called for extra money to go into the social care system where the needs are greatest (Bosch, 2021).

Away from the pressure cooker of acute hospitals, primary care and community health staff are struggling too, which undermines efforts to help people to remain at home instead of ending up in an ambulance, hospital or care home. The number of social care staff had fallen by at least 42,000 in the six months to the end of October 2021, but the true loss is more likely to be between 50,000 and 70,000 (Oung, 2021). By November 2021, 400,000 people were waiting for their care needs to be assessed and for care to be provided. One and a half million hours of home care could not be covered because of insufficient staff, despite record amounts of home care being provided (ADASS, 2021b). Plans to extend the 'no jab, no job' policy to home care workers will have led, by the government's own estimates, to a further 35,000 staff leaving the sector (DHSC, 2021d). These losses could have been avoided, as the government later decided to reverse the policy. By January 2022, the regulator was reporting that vacancy rates had doubled since the previous April to over 11 per cent and that staff turnover in care homes had reached 36 per cent (Care Quality Commission, 2022).

Behind these big figures lie other failings that attract only fleeting publicity. In December 2021 Tony Hickmott, aged 44, was still languishing in an assessment and treatment unit where he has lived since 2002, longer than he has ever lived in his own home. He was declared 'fit for discharge' in 2013, but was held up because of wrangles between the NHS and the local council about sorting out his care needs. Tony is one of a hundred people with learning disabilities and autism who have been in specialist hospitals for at least 20 years. For the almost 2,000 people in England who live in these places, the institutions never went away (BBC News, 2021b). There are countless others who need care and support in places like prisons and hostels for homeless people, in drug and alcohol rehabilitation units, on the streets and other places that are less likely to attract the positive gaze of the public than the venerated NHS and those considered to be 'deserving'.

The problems afflicting social care are now so serious, extensive and deep-seated that reforms that merely seek to ameliorate the existing system will almost certainly fail. The oft-overlooked orphan of the UK welfare state, social care is scarred by decades of underfunding, fragmentation, poor commissioning and short-term sticking plasters that have drained its resilience and capacity to rise to the challenge of changing needs, modern aspirations and the potential of technology. For too many people, the 'system' is difficult to understand, access to the right kind of support is very limited and hard to attain and involves very high costs. On top of these old problems, that were there long before COVID-19, are piled the newer challenges of an increasingly depleted and exhausted workforce, fresh demands arising from long COVID and other pandemic sequela, dealing with the backlog of unmet need and managing the uncertain consequences of new coronavirus variants.

All of these demands are mounting up faster than the current ability of politicians and governments to respond to them. Held up against the mirror of these challenges, the measures proposed to deal with them fall well short of the plan promised by the prime minister that would fix the crisis in social care 'once and for all.' As they stand, the government's proposals resemble a dead end rather than a road map for reform. They neither tackle head-on the immediate pressures nor amount to a long-term plan. Indeed, there is a real risk that the government's proposals for a cap on care costs will unravel, like the Dilnot proposals in 2015, as the financial squeeze on councils intensifies in the months ahead and political opposition to the National Insurance rise stiffens in response to mounting pressures on household finances. By February 2022, the Local Government Association was warning that under-resourcing could derail the government's funding reforms, destabilise existing services and leave the public paying more through higher taxes for less care (Local Government Association, 2022). Although polling carried out in November and December 2021 suggests the public appear to support the new health and social care levy, nearly two-thirds do not think the government has the right policies for social care and most are pessimistic about the future (Buzelli et al, 2022).

Instead, the crisis is deepening, driven by multiple and profound weaknesses that speak to a need for an entirely different model of social care; one based not on making the existing system work better, but replacing it with something very different and far more ambitious. The time for improvement alone has passed.

The economic and social case for care

Across the Atlantic, there is another version of 'Build Back Better' that could not be more different from the UK government's version. In November 2021, the House of Representatives passed legislation of that name to rebuild the US economy and strengthen its social safety net. It included $400 billion to create jobs and improve the pay and conditions of home care workers, 'the majority of whom are women of color and … have been underpaid and undervalued for too long', and providing home and community-based care for people who otherwise would have had to wait as long as five years (White House, 2021). This version of 'Build Back Better' stands out from the UK version by virtue of the sheer scale of the proposed investment and the coupling of social justice and economic need, framed as 'improving the infrastructure of the care economy' (Congressional Budget Office, 2021).

The USA is not the first country most experts would look to for a model of good long-term care. The bill faces formidable obstacles to get through Senate and has already been scaled back considerable to get this far. But President Biden's plans illustrate that if bold and big thinking can emerge in such a deeply inauspicious political climate, why should it not be possible to apply a similar level of ambition and imagination in tackling the problems of social care in England? To apply the Irish proverb to the common analogy of social care reform as a journey, we would not want to start from here, reacting to a deepening crisis that inevitably takes us down a path of yet more short-term initiatives that rarely deliver what they promise.

Drawing on the conclusions of the previous chapter, a completely different road to reform is possible, resting on twin foundational principles of social and economic wellbeing. Social care represents a huge force for good in society and makes a difference every day to many hundreds of thousands of lives throughout the land. Too often, this happens despite the system not because of it. It is rarely made possible by the great armadas of White Papers, commissions or think tank reports, although they do have a part to play, but by a far bigger flotilla of much smaller ships in local places. This is in communities, through voluntary groups, care providers and the millions of people, paid and unpaid, who help people to lead a better life, sometimes at times of great distress or crisis. When the right kind of support is available, at the right time and in the right place, with the individual in the driving seat, social care can and does change lives, as some of the testimony in this book attests.

Changing demographics and structures of family life mean that social care is rapidly becoming a universal concern for most of us, not just a minority of people traditionally labelled as vulnerable and different. One of the lessons to be learned from other countries (discussed in Chapter 5) is how public support for change can be achieved by emphasising the benefits of good care to people and their families. It includes the peace of mind made possible by better, reliable access to good-quality support, without recourse to the language of warfare used by many people to describe their struggle to get help. In the 1940s, Nye Bevan described the 'serenity' that would come from access to good medical care through the NHS without financial or other barriers. The appreciation of that quality has powered the high levels of public and political support that has sustained the NHS for over 70 years. There is no reason why this cannot be extended to social care if its benefits and potential can be communicated and understood in the same way.

The case for social care as a force for economic wellbeing is also strong. In 2020–21 it added £25.6 billion of GVA (the gross value added to England's economy by the goods and services it produces). This rises to £50.3 billion when direct and indirect benefits are added in. These multiplier effects are important in social care because a relatively-low-paid workforce will spend a much higher proportion of their pay on other goods and services that boost the wider economy. If the government intends to 'level up' those parts of the country that have been left behind economically, investing in social care is a good tool to use. Adult social care accounted for 1.6 per cent of the country's GVA in 2020–21. That might sound a small percentage, but in these terms it is a bigger sector than electricity and power, water and waste management, and twice as big as agriculture. Because demand for social care is relatively predictable, shaped as it is by long-term demographic trends, higher spending could help to stabilise the ups and downs of the business cycle in the wider economy. The sector is growing too, with the number of jobs increasing, compared with falling employment in other sectors. Further economic benefits could be secured through spending more on social care. Of working-age people with care needs, 57 per cent are able to work if offered the right support to do so. Better support for unpaid carers would enable them to return to employment or make it easier to hold down existing jobs (Skills for Care and KD Network Analytics, 2021). Offering more support to unpaid carers also boosts their wellbeing (Forder, 2018).

In the USA, the movement Across the Generations has achieved some success in shaping the 'Build Back Better' legislation by arguing that the future of work and the future of care are inextricably linked. Its proposition that a modern economy needs a transport infrastructure of bridges, buses, trains and roads so people can get to work is hardly controversial. But people need care to get to work, too, whether that is access to child care or help for their older or disabled relatives. At both ends of the generational spectrum, a good social infrastructure is as important as the physical infrastructure.

As well as missing the benefits of good care, inadequate investment in social care creates costs and externalities in other spheres of life. Cuts in care spending since 2010 are associated with big increases in the use of emergency hospital care by older people (Crawford et al, 2021). Recent analysis of the relationship between health and social care spending and mortality rates indicates that additional social care spending is more than twice as productive in saving lives as is additional health care expenditure (Martin et al, 2021). Just a fraction of the 40 per cent real-term funding boost to the NHS since 2010 could have had a much bigger impact had it been diverted to social care. People being stuck in hospital while waiting for an assessment, or help so they can go home, results in significant human and financial costs. Then there is the impact of low pay in social care, and lack of support for unpaid carers, on gender inequality and the economic and social consequences that flow from this. Gender gaps in the labour market are known to dent economic growth. Instead of contributing to gender inequalities, action to raise the status and pay levels in social care and to support unpaid carers to hold down jobs would help to reverse them. Ironically, under existing measures of output, a woman who looks after a partner or relative is deemed to contribute nothing to national wealth, whereas, if she were paid to do so, the value of that care would be counted (Andrew et al, 2021). Social care is not well served by traditional measures of productivity and GDP. There is a bigger debate here, beyond the scope of this book, about what we mean by economic value, the activities that create wealth rather than extract from it, and the potential to develop better measures of the things that are important to us (Mazzucato, 2018).

So, there is a wide range of benefits to society and the economy from seeing social care spending not as a cost centre or a drain on the nation's wealth, but as a dynamic engine of economic and social wellbeing. This is especially so in those parts of the country that have been left behind economically and are the focus of the government's levelling-up strategy. There are some key lessons to be learned, outlined in Chapter 5, from those countries that have successfully introduced reforms to long-term care by focusing on longer range economic and social benefits instead of reacting to the immediate crisis of the moment. The economic benefits of state spending on education and health care in securing a healthy and educated workforce were recognised long before the creation of the British welfare state. The acknowledgement of similar benefits for social care spending is long overdue.

The sweet spot when those economic and social benefits of social care are combined to produce great outcomes for people and for society is illustrated by the story of Abbie, who has cerebral palsy. The right kind of support through a personal assistant meant that she could obtain a university degree, get a job, and enjoy family life. Her words are another reminder of the importance of reciprocity and interdependence in thinking about how to design a better care system:

> My husband and children will care for me, but they
> are not my carers. I don't want them to be. While

> I get PA support from somebody I trust, I hope I can love and care for my husband and children as much as they love and care for me. That's all I ever wanted out of life. (Skills for Care and KD Network Analytics, 2021)

Looking at the case for social care investment through a different lens brings into focus the much bigger 'social care pound', outlined in Chapter 3. Policy-makers have traditionally concentrated on what local authorities spend as the be-all-and end-all of social care. Lamentations about underfunding and austerity overlook the much bigger resources tied up in other public funding streams, private spending and the resources of the voluntary sector and communities – the notion of the social care pound. Irrespective of how much it spends, the state could be a much smarter spender. How could this massive, combined resource be moulded imaginatively to produce better outcomes for people?

One example is the way social security benefits for older and disabled people operate entirely separately from the social care system. Disability groups have understandably been suspicious of ideas that would see their entitlement to financial benefits, aimed at income support needs, sucked into a rationed and cash-strapped social care system. As it is, too many are lost to social care charges. But there is no reason why existing entitlements to attendance allowance (a cash benefit payable by the DWP to people over 65 years old with care needs) could not be rebranded. As a care and support allowance and promoted more widely as a universal benefit, not means-tested or taxed, it would help to foster wellbeing (Commission on the Future of Health and Social Care in England, 2014a).

Although several governments have urged local councils and their partners to share their resources, through initiatives like Total Place, community budgets and place-based commissioning, they have preferred to urge it from others rather than practise it themselves. Certainly, it would be tricky, complicated work, hindered by those keen to protect their own budget silos, and it would take far too long for the usual transitory here-today, gone-tomorrow time horizons of policy-makers. The ability of local government, the NHS and other public services to bend and align their budgets towards better outcomes for local people, rather than narrow organisational objectives, will be one of the biggest challenges for England's fledging integrated care systems (Ham, 2022).

A universal service – and its limits

There are compelling arguments for social care to be placed centre stage as a major public service in its own right, not a shadowy adjunct to the NHS or the forgotten Cinderella of the post-war welfare state. It cannot be emphasised often enough that the necessity of having a good social care system is not a response to failure, but a consequence of the success story of rising living standards, the capacity of modern health care to help us live longer lives and the countless possibilities of scientific and technological advance. It is not simply about adding years to lives, but adding life to those additional years. We will want quality lives, not just longer lives, which is the core purpose of social care. A powerful argument for a universal approach arises from the likelihood that most of us will need some kind of care and support at some point in our lives, while the nature, cost and duration of those needs remains unpredictable.

The economic and social case for a new, comprehensive and universal approach to social care rests in part on its interdependence with other areas of economic and social policy. The benefits of good care are wide-ranging, but there are limits to what social care on can achieve on its own. It is now well accepted that the NHS, on its own, cannot make it possible for people to lead healthy lives. That depends on wider determinants of health, such as income, education, housing, transport and leisure, the physical environment, relationships with friends and family, as well as genetics and lifestyle choices. Social care is a poor and expensive response to the problems of loneliness. The relatively new concept of population health is about moving away from a system just focused on diagnosing and treating illness towards one that is based on promoting wellbeing and preventing ill health. This is not just down to the NHS, but is a responsibility shared with a host of national and local bodies, those working with local communities, and, of course, individuals themselves (Buck et al, 2018). A good example is the work of Care City, a community interest company in East London that works across health and social care to promote healthy ageing and community regeneration (Craig, 2021).

The same arguments apply in abundance to social care. Physical and mental health issues are among the most common reasons why people need social care. Anything that helps reduces the number of people with long-term health conditions, or helps them to manage an existing condition better, is likely to reduce their need for care and support. The importance of good primary care and community health services in supporting people to live as independently as possible for as long as possible is crucial to making that happen. The problems inadequate social care causes for the NHS, such as avoidable use of emergency care or people stuck in hospital waiting for care at home are very well-publicised. But it is not a one-way street. Weaknesses in basic health care provision, such as district nursing, podiatry, chiropody, physiotherapy and occupational therapy, can cause older people with multiple chronic illnesses to end up in long-term care (Bolton, 2016). There is an abundance of evidence about the value of integrated health and social care to prevent, limit or postpone dependency on long-term care services (Oliver et al, 2014).

Older and disabled people who live in warm, well-insulated and appropriately designed housing are less likely to become ill and need either medical or social help (Garrett et al, 2021). People of all ages who live in communities that are safe and thriving, where neighbours look out for each other, with a vibrant social infrastructure of community groups, clubs, faith groups and pubs are more likely to lead happier lives. Working-age people with disabilities who are helped to get and hold down a job will lead a better life than those at home all day, or where the only option for something to do or somewhere to go, is a day centre. Although the pension triple lock has helped to lift the value of the state pension, poverty and income inequality remains higher than the average in OECD countries (OECD, 2021a). So, although it is impossible to disagree with the #SocialCareFuture vision of how 'we all want to live in the place we call home, be with the people and things that we love and do the things that matter to us, in communities where we all care about and support each other' (Crowther, 2020), those conditions cannot be created by a formal, state-run social care system alone. We should not expect more of publicly organised and funded social care than we do of God.

A precondition for effective social care is a range of parallel public policies, particularly in areas like pensions and benefits, housing, community development and criminal justice. Deficits in these other parts of the public service landscape have prompted many health and care organisations to devise particular solutions, such as social prescribing or asset-based community development (Social Care Institute for Excellence, 2017). These are welcome, but their potential can be compromised by being framed in clinical language as a response to deficits, or re-inventions of what councils used to do through their community development functions in the 1970s and 1980. Rather, they could be seen as part of the general infrastructure of local community resources available to all, as they are in some places, instead of annexed to the cause of specific groups or individuals deemed to be needy, disadvantaged or vulnerable.

Social care both depends on and contributes to a thriving economy that offers good jobs and generates higher tax revenues to pay for good public services, including social care. The wider social infrastructure of communities, by making it easier for people to lead a good life, will help to reduce the need for formal services. The general point here is that the focus of analysis is too often on the numbers and costs of people entering the formal care system. Less attention is paid to considering how well a range of public policies more generally is enabling older and disabled people to achieve the best life possible. A useful tool is the Active Ageing Index, developed by the United Nations Economic Commission for Europe, that measures the extent to which older and disabled people can realise their full potential in terms of employment and participation in social and cultural life, and independent living (United Nations, 2019).

By positioning social care as an integral feature of England's social and economic infrastructure, it becomes possible to imagine a very different approach to care and support, comprising three interlinked building blocks – a new social contract; a redesigned model of care and support; and a new long-term funding settlement.

The ties that bind – a new social contract

All societies are based on a set of views about what aspects of life should be left to individuals and what should be the responsibility of the state. Or, as Minouche Shafik puts it, 'How much *does* society owe an individual and how much does the individual owe society?' (Shafik, 2021). This in turn requires judgements about the benefits that can be secured by individuals only through collective solidarity. The implicit social contract of the post-war welfare state promised universal health care, family allowances, basic national assistance, pensions and education. In return for the largesse of these universal provisions, people (or, to be more precise, male breadwinners) were expected to go to work and pay their taxes. Based on life expectancy at the time, it was thought that most retirees would not be claiming their pension for long. The default assumption was that wives would stay at home to care for children and dependent adults. The social contract of the 1940s is now irredeemably broken on the wheel of demography, changing patterns of employment and family life and the rising volume, acuity and complexity of care needs.

The consequences for social care of remaining trapped within its tramlines have been dire. Responsibilities for providing care are now borne mostly on the shoulders of individuals and families, usually women, who are expected to work and care. The basic safety net offered by the state has become increasingly threadbare. The proposed cap on care costs will, if implemented, extend the state's offer, but relatively few people will benefit. It will remain the case that, while the very poorest will receive care free at the point of use (though at some cost to their financial benefits) and the richest will easily pay for themselves, everyone in the middle is expected to bear the financial risk with little support. Many continue to labour under the illusion that social care costs will be taken care of by the NHS. If everyone were aware of just how lopsided the existing social contract is, it is hard to imagine that anyone would choose to sign it.

The absence of an explicit social contract has also led to some piecemeal workarounds that have sought to bolster the contribution of communities rather than the state. This includes ideas about a 'big society' and the emergence of new asset-based approaches that aim to strengthen the resilience of communities and their capacity to find their own solutions to supporting people. At one level, these are laudable, but in the context of a decade of austerity in public services from 2010, they run the risk of dumping problems on councils, care providers and individuals. The state has also stealthily shunted more of the costs of care towards local taxpayers and self-funders. The converse proposition that all care should be the responsibility of the state is equally inappropriate and financially unsustainable.

Other countries have developed very different kinds of social contracts for care. Nordic countries, for example, offer generous public services in return for high levels of taxation. The social insurance models adopted by many countries offer a different type of social contact that offers guaranteed levels of entitlement to care, but requires mandatory contributions from individuals and employers.

The social contract is not simply between individual citizens and the state. There are important issues about the contributions of individuals to their local communities and particularly their role in supporting its members with care needs. There is some evidence that, in the years before COVID came, there had been a decline in social capital (covering such things as contact with neighbours, helping out older and disabled people and engagement with the local community) and that 'we are engaging less with our neighbours but more with social media' (ONS, 2020). The pandemic has thrown into sharp relief how much we depend on each other and the mutual benefits that flow from sharing risks and making sacrifices; benefits that cannot be achieved by individuals on their own. It is too soon to say how much the resurgence of mutual support and volunteering will reverse the decline in social capital.

Either way, it underlines the importance of a new social contract that is less about 'me' and more about 'we' (Shafik,

2021). Rather than being confined to the relationship between the individual and the state, it could lay out a broader matrix of the rights, responsibilities and mutual obligations of people and communities, local and central government, as well as the intermediate layer of voluntary and other bodies. Such a contract should cover comprehensively a wide range of entitlements and obligations, from income support to work and taxation, education, child care, employment and democratic participation. That is clearly beyond the scope of this book, which concentrates on rights and responsibilities for care and support.

A new 21st-century social contract for care, sitting within a wider social contract, is now long overdue as one of the essential building blocks of a new approach to social care. For many years, people with care and support needs have been treated as dependent, vulnerable clients reliant on the state to have their needs met. Later on, the community care reforms in the 1990s tried to reposition them as consumers, exercising choice and control in a marketplace of competing providers (Hudson, 2021). Later still, efforts to give people more rights, for example through the Care Act 2014 or through human rights legislation, have floundered through a mixture of legal inexactitude and austerity. A new social contract instead could be based on a citizenship model, setting out the mutual rights as well as the obligations we owe to each other as fellow citizens, whether we give or receive care and support, noting that at different points of our lives we will do either or sometimes both.

Older people might be expected to work longer, reflecting their longer lives, in return for greater security in later life: a commitment that they will get the support they need to live as independently as possible in their own homes. Responsibilities for care that currently sit overwhelmingly with women could shift to one shared with society, so that better support for carers would reduce gender inequalities. This has the potential to improve the quality of women's lives and enable them to contribute to the economy and society through paid employment or in other ways. The term used by the Japanese government when it launched its long-term care insurance scheme was 'From Care by Family to Care by Society'. In a similar vein, better support for people with disabilities would enable them to contribute to society through employment and paying taxes. Making it easier for people to contribute to society in a variety of ways ought to be key component of any new social contract, reinforcing Amartya Sen's arguments for a 'capability' approach in which individuals are offered not merely a basic minimum of provision but what they need to help them realise their aspirations (Sen, 1999). Reciprocity, not care dependency, needs to be the driving principle behind a new approach.

A new social contract could speak to concerns about intergenerational fairness in how care is paid for. It could do this by making explicit the reality that most of us already pay more into the system, via taxes, during our working lives, and we take out most, via public services and benefits, in the earlier part of our lives (through child care and education) and in later years (through pensions, health and social care), illustrated in Figure 8.1.

Already, the boundaries between the three traditional life stages of childhood and education, adulthood and employment and old age and retirement are set to become more blurred in response to longevity and changes in the world of work. These shifts make it even more important to encourage everyone to give and receive reciprocally at different stages of life instead of fretting about the perceived unfairness between generations that has distorted the 'who pays' question about social care. There is also a social contract between this generation and future ones that reinforces the argument for a long-term approach to social care reform and cathedral thinking.

A new social contract for care cannot be imposed through legislation and guidance from above. There are different views about where the balance should sit in a new matrix of rights and responsibilities that criss-cross the roles of central and local government, civil society and individuals, families and communities. The choices and trade-offs are intrinsically political. They are less about analysis and evidence (though this supplies the raw materials for the debate), and more about values and priorities. The options are not straightforward, and the difficulties of reaching consensus should not be underestimated. The best answers about how social care should be reformed are not necessarily what some believe to be the right answers

Figure 8.1: Age profile of public spending and tax

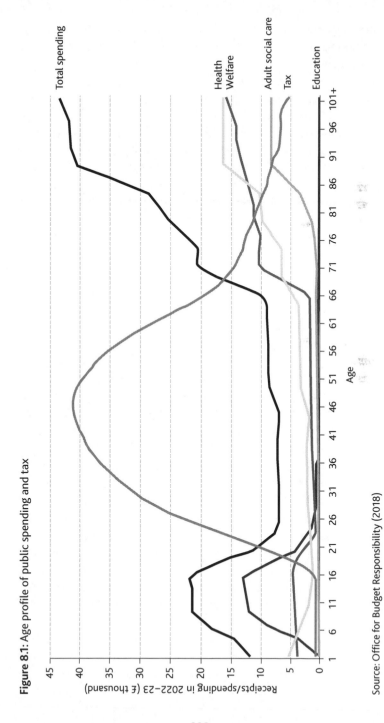

Source: Office for Budget Responsibility (2018)

but the ones that command the most support. It cannot be left to the hothouse of Westminster politics, with predictable consequences. Instead, echoing Overton's point about convincing voters rather than politicians, the debate could be taken directly to the public, through a fundamentally different approach to policy-making, as proposed in the previous chapter. A different national conversation and debate, built upwards from many local ones, could help to raise public awareness of the benefits of good care and support to individuals, families and the economy. For the first time, this could move us towards a shared understanding, if not a consensus, about the balance of rights and responsibilities in providing and paying for care. And it could help embolden parliamentarians and policy-makers to grasp the nettle.

Subject to that process, what might a new social contract for care look like? A starting point is that incremental improvements will not be enough and that a profound reset is required. Some of the big ideas that could be put forward include:

Enshrining in law the right of people of all ages to live independently in their own homes. This is the preference of the overwhelming majority of people, with some evidence that it has strengthened because of COVID-19 (Ilinca, 2021). Article 19 of the United Nations Convention on the Rights of Persons with Disabilities (UNCRPD), to which the UK is a signatory, sets out the rights of disabled people to live independently, including the right to choose where to live. But this has never been incorporated into UK law (United Nations, 2007 and 2017). Existing human rights, equality and community care laws fail to achieve it. A new right to independent living, applying to people of all ages, would, if accompanied by other changes, decisively shift the whole character of social care from a discretionary, eligibility-determined assessment process towards a rights-based entitlement. It could bring alive the original Care Act aspirations to promote wellbeing. But, to be meaningful, it would depend on an adequate funding settlement and new arrangements for implementation and enforcement of these rights as part of a new delivery model for social care, discussed later.

Creating a universal offer from the state, covering advice and information, assessment, prevention, good housing and basic universal health care and a basic minimum income for all, as part of a wider social contract, is a prerequisite for individual and community wellbeing. It is important to note too that the concept of independent living involves participating in society as a full and equal citizen and underscores the importance of the wider social contract in which these ideas are positioned.

Being clear about how much good care costs and how this should be paid for, accepting that the benefits of good care can be secured only through comprehensive risk-pooling through either general taxation or social insurance. This could include options for people to use their own private wealth to lead better lives, with everyone enjoying protection from catastrophic costs. It should include protecting working-age disabled people from losing a significant chunk of their benefits to care charges. How care is paid for is a central pillar of a new social contract and should form the basis of a new funding settlement discussed later.

Acknowledging the reciprocal responsibilities of individuals to contribute towards the wellbeing of their communities. A new social contract should not just be a transactional agreement with the state but also reflect what we owe to each other, our fellow citizens. These contributions could take many forms. The obvious one is contributing financially, according to our individual means, to the costs of a much more generous and comprehensive entitlement to care and support, through local and national taxation or co-payment. But there are other significant contributions people can make 'in kind', through voluntary work, membership of a local group, offering unpaid care or simply being a good neighbour, underlining again the importance of reciprocity and mutuality in our relationships with each other.

Accepting our responsibilities towards our family and loved ones needing care and support, in the knowledge that we can access timely and effective help from public services without being expected to shoulder the responsibilities of caring on our own, especially where care needs are intense and all-consuming. This would mean a new deal for unpaid carers with a range of measures, including an adequate carer's allowance, access to respite care and support at home, and other incentives and support to enable carers to enter and remain in the labour market.

A wider social contract could also *encourage and support people to pursue a healthy lifestyle*, possibly with financial and other incentives, that enables a better quality of life and lessens the need to use health and care services. It might even extend to a moral, if not legal, obligation to be vaccinated against infectious and life-threatening diseases.

The aim here is to reconnect people's expectations of social care with the means to achieve them at a national level. There is no reason why, at the level of 'place', social care leaders could not try to develop their own local framework of expectations with local residents and people with care and support needs. These local conversations could then feed into national deliberations about a new contract for care. The best-known example, led by local government, is Wigan, which has tried to transform the way it delivers its services and develop a different approach to meeting needs. In the face of rising demand and reducing resources, the essence of what has come to be known as 'the Wigan Deal' is that, in return for the council keeping the council tax as low as possible and providing appropriate services, the residents of Wigan would do their bit by recycling more, getting involved in the community and trying to stay fit and healthy (Figure 8.2). It has been described as a 'give–get' agreement between the council and local people (Naylor and Wellings, 2019).

A new design and delivery model

The problems with the way England's existing social care system is structured and organised have been well-documented in previous chapters. The underlying causes include the fragmentation of responsibilities between 151 councils and over 19,000 independent providers; commissioning approaches driven by costs rather than outcomes for people; hand-to-mouth funding; and chronic workforce shortages. To many, it appears to be a system driven by the needs of organisations rather than

Figure 8.2: The Deal between Wigan Council and local people

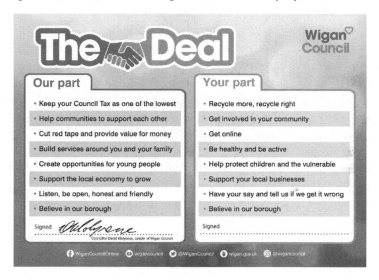

Source: Naylor and Wellings (2019)

the people they are supposed to serve. There have been many examples of ideas and innovation, usually from care providers and local initiatives, that led to people getting better support (Think Local Act Personal, 2018), but commissioners have struggled to scale these up, to be available everywhere, and scale down traditional services that demonstrably fail to meet needs (Sanders, 2021). Tinkering with existing arrangements will not be enough. Much bigger changes are needed to the way social care works and to overcome resistance to change. These could include:

Placing more power in the hands of people to shape their care and support arrangements. For many years, the default operating model for social care has involved personal budgets, culminating in the Care Act 2014. Yet the rhetoric of self-directed support, with personalisation too often conflated with giving people a lump of money, has not been translated into reality. Despite their almost universal popularity and the evidence of how they can change lives, fewer people than ever are opting for direct payments, with concerns about the restrictive and controlling way some councils are implementing them (Think Local Act

Personal, 2021). The odds are stacked against people having the right to choose how, and by whom, their personal budget should be managed, so, this should be bolstered by a new right to independent advocacy and practical support to help manage a direct payment.

Establishing a new network of independent advisory centres to offer advice, information and brokerage to help people get the right support. This would help to ensure that new rights to independent living and self-direct support can be enforced. These new centres could employ independent social workers, financial advisors and housing options advisors. They would offer support workers to help people to manage the personal budget they have chosen. Each local centre, which could be built from existing centres for independent living, could be required to collaborate through regional and networks so that specialist legal and other advice is available. Crucially, they should have sufficient teeth and resources to help individuals exercise their rights to independent living, through advocacy, mediation and, if necessary legal challenge.

Launching an ambitious Home is Best programme to pump-prime a decisive shift in the balance of resources from acute hospital and long-term care facilities towards care at home. A joint endeavour with the NHS, it would be funded through a five-year, multi-billion-pound transformation fund, ring-fenced for care and support at home. Embracing health and housing as well as social care needs, local partnerships would agree how the grant should be deployed, delivered and monitored. Depending on local needs, priorities for investment might include new rapid response teams to avoid hospital admissions, investments to stimulate local community-based capacity, adaptations to property, integrated care-at-home teams such as Buurtzorg, assistive technology and home care support (see, for example, British Geriatrics Society, 2021). The success of this Home is Best programme could be judged by the number of people supported to live at home and the reduction in the use of acute hospital and long-term residential care.

Implementing major reforms to the current 'market' in social care. In the same way that the NHS is moving away from a purchaser–provider split, there are compelling arguments for replacing conventional contracting models in social care based largely on price with a collaborative model that encourages councils and providers to innovate. Success should be measured primarily by the outcomes achieved, not just by activities and costs. This would mean a rebalancing of existing services towards local, not-for-profit organisations that are rooted in their local communities and achieve better quality and outcomes than larger, distant corporate entities (Fox, 2018; Hudson, 2021). Some have called for the nationalisation of privately owned care services, but this would be legally arduous, take too long and cost too much, without any immediate benefit to the people who use them. In any case the key issue here is not ownership per se but transparency of financing, the size of facilities and how close they are to local communities, and the quality of its leadership and workforce. A better starting point would be to tackle the most egregious excesses of what Jeremy Hunt has called 'the unacceptable face of capitalism' – very large, private-equity funded corporate care home providers with complex and opaque business models, high levels of debt and the extraction of money to private investors in offshore tax havens (Melley and Holt, 2021; CICTAR, 2021). One estimate suggests that around £1.5 billion leaks out of the care home industry annually in the form of rent, dividend payments, net interest payments, directors' fees and profits before tax. Leakage rates for the largest providers are almost double those of the smallest ones (Kotecha, 2019). As was noted in Chapter 3, the incursion of private finance into public care, almost by stealth, is an inevitable consequence of the state's effective withdrawal from investing in new services and facilities. As well as a new public funding settlement to reverse this, new controls are needed to ensure greater transparency in where care home income goes, and tighter business regulation of companies who are allowed to provide care in the UK.

Balancing investment in care at home with high-quality residential care where this is the right option. COVID-19 has understandably heightened concerns about the risks and appropriateness of congregate living for older and disabled people, including the impact on their physical and psychological health of restrictions on visiting and access to health care. The major expansion of home care and a strengthened right to independent living proposed earlier, if implemented well, should reduce the *proportion* of people in residential care. But projections are clear that the overall *numbers* of people with very high levels of care need are set to grow substantially by 2030 (Kingston et al, 2018a). As Andrea Sutcliffe, a former chief inspector of social care, observed in 2018, there will be a continuing need for some kind of residential care, particularly nursing homes for people with the extensive, complex needs: 'However much an individual, their family or the community would want to support people to live and die in their own homes', she observed, 'sometimes this just won't be possible for a whole host of reasons' (Sutcliffe, 2018). The key question, therefore, is what is the best model, or models, of congregate living, in terms of personal acceptability, design, size, costs and ownership? Creative thinking is needed about a range of group living options, including boutique care home models, extra-care and retirement housing, co-housing and supported living schemes (Social Care Institute for Excellence, 2021). The aim should be to expand options and choices instead of reducing the issue to a binary one of 'residential care = bad; home and community care = good.'

Gradually aligning entitlement to social care with that of health care, initially by making high levels of personal care free at the point of use. This would virtually end the division between means-tested social care and continuing healthcare that has imposed heavy human as well as financial costs on those caught up in it. This echoes a key recommendation of the Barker Commission in 2014 (Commission on the Future of Health and Social Care in England, 2014a). Whether the entitlement to social care could be further universalised in this way would depend on preferences and choices arising from a new social contract and a funding settlement to support it.

A different role for local authorities. The shift towards a stronger rights-led ethos would see council block-commissioning of care gradually displaced by most people making their own care and support arrangements, with support from the new independent advisory centres. The role of councils would change from negotiating and contracting with providers towards strategically planning for the needs of their local population as a whole. In future, councils would work collaboratively with providers to promote innovation and oversee the coordination and development of services across the whole public service landscape. Although much of this work will be done at the level of 'place', there is a crucial role here for councils in giving voice to the cause of individual and community wellbeing in the bigger geographical footprint of the new Integrated Care Systems and Integrated Health and Care Partnerships (Charles, 2021). It is important that councils are held to account for their part in ensuring that people get good social care. The new assurance arrangements the government is planning to introduce to monitor councils' performance should concentrate on how well outcomes are being achieved, for both individuals and communities.

Implementing major reforms to enhance the pay, status and training of the social care workforce. There can be no solution to England's social care crisis without a sweeping and ambitious ten-year people plan, drawing on some of the ideas put forward in Chapter 6. A thread running through this book is the centrality of people in social care, not just in terms of the numbers needed, but in nurturing the quality of relationships between those giving and receiving care through decent pay and a good infrastructure for training, support and career progression. This could include planning a renaissance in the trinity of regulated professions in social care – social work, nursing and occupational therapy – whose specialist skills will be needed more than ever in the years ahead (see, for example, Royal College of Occupational Therapists, 2021).

A new funding settlement

Finally, the thorniest set of questions of all concern how we pay for the care and support we need. Many people have pointed out that better social care is not just about money, which is why it is the final building block to be considered in this final chapter.

In absolute terms, the figures look large. The government has already pledged an extra £5.4 billion for social care over the next three years, through the new health and social care levy. Most of this will pay for a new cap on care costs, a more generous means test and bringing council rates for residential care in line with what self-funders pay. There is little left to meet rising demand, tackling unmet needs or enabling providers to boost staff wages. These pressures would require further additional funding of around £7.6 billion in 2022–23, rising to £9.0bn in 2024–25 (Tallack et al, 2021). Further steps to make social care more universal, for example by providing more care free at the point of use, and a new Home is Best programme, proposed earlier, would swell further the overall costs of social care.

But there are some important caveats about these numbers. They start from a low baseline, characterised by a mean means test, falling spending in real terms and fewer people getting help. Adult social care accounted for less than 4 per cent of all state spending on public services in England in 2019–20. This ratio is completely out of kilter with the country's need for an economic and social infrastructure that provides good well-paid jobs and helps people – carers and cared for – to contribute to society. It is unavoidable that any serious attempt to move away from the current system, which rations help only to those with the highest needs and lowest means, towards a more universal footing that we take for granted as for other services such as education and health care, will come with a hefty price tag.

Making progress on the funding issue has been hindered by a misconception that the costs of care can be avoided or ducked. It is inevitable that the country will spend more on social care as the population grows and ages. The question is not whether more money is spent, but where the costs will fall. The current trend is for them to fall to individuals – council-tax-payers rather than central government. They do so in a haphazard, arbitrary way that is not widely understand and makes it impossible for both the public bodies involved and individuals and families to plan ahead. And it does not make sense for the NHS to continue its trajectory of absorbing an ever-bigger share of day-to-day government spending – 46 per cent by 2024–25 (Tallack et al, 2021) – without commensurate increases for social care, given their interdependency.

Then there is the argument that spending large sums of money on social care is unaffordable, a notion that surely has been undermined completely by the explosion in public spending triggered by COVID-19. Since the pandemic took hold, the government has found at least £155 billion of new funding to help public services respond to the crisis (Institute for Government, 2021a). At one point in the crisis, for example, the Test and Trace budget was suddenly boosted by £7 billion, roughly the same as spending on social care for older people, with a total budget on a par with social care spending on people of all ages. In words attributed to the late US senator Everett Dirksen, 'A billion here, a billion there, and pretty soon you're talking real money' (United States Senate, 1969). All spending choices by governments are the product of judgements not about whether something can be afforded in an absolute sense, but its relative priority set against other spending.

The Health Foundation has calculated that a £12-billion per annum investment package for social care, including a generous £46,000 cap on care costs, works out at just 0.4 per cent of GDP. The cap element would cost the equivalent of £2.14 per household per week, just under what households spend on buildings and contents insurance. The extra cost of the bigger element of the spending package would be £5.95 per week per household, just under half of average weekly spending on car insurance (Charlesworth et al, 2021). The public are generally unaware of these comparisons because they have never been allowed the opportunity to contribute to a discussion about the choices and trade-offs between them. That is why it so essential to shift the debate from the corridors of Whitehall and Westminster and expose the issues to the sunlight of open, public debate.

The fairest and most effective way of dealing with the risks of social care is by sharing them as widely as possible across the whole population, through taxation or mandatory social insurance (Nuffield Trust, 2019). This is how we fund the NHS, and many countries have adopted universal risk-pooling as the central funding mechanism for long-term care as well as health care (as set out in Chapter 4). Mandatory public funding would therefore be the predominant funding source for social care. Using taxation would be simpler to understand, easy to administer through the existing tax system and be relatively fair in that one-third of income tax is paid by the richest 1 per cent of the population. Introducing mandatory social insurance would strengthen people's entitlements to a defined level of care, but the downside is that it would require new administrative systems and processes. Because people's contributions could only be used for social care, it introduces inflexibility that could undermine the funding of other public services on which social care is dependent. Ring-fencing (hypothecation) works well for services that the public know and like, less so for those they do not. One outcome of the social contract debate might be that people are prepared to pay more for social care, but only if assured that the money will be spent solely on social care and accompanied by a guaranteed entitlement (see, for example, Ipsos Mori 2018 and 2021). Compulsory social insurance might be the sugar on the pill that policy-makers need to swallow to secure the scale of funding needed.

A mixture of funding sources will almost certainly be required over time. Countries with well-established social insurance systems have needed to supplement this through general taxation and adjusting individual contributions and out-of-pocket charges to balance overall funding with rising needs and costs (Cylus et al, 2018). There are various permutations of how money could be raised by changing tax rates and allowances, bearing in mind that most money is raised by income tax, National Insurance and VAT. For illustrative purposes, a simple one percentage point increase on each of these taxes in 2023–24 would generate the following amounts:

- basic and higher rate of income tax: £6.6 billion;
- National Insurance Class 1 employee main rate: £4 billion;
- National Insurance Class 1 employer main rate: £7.4 billion;
- VAT at standard rate: £7. 5 billion (HM Revenue and Customs, 2021).

The options for how social care could be funded have been examined exhaustively (for example by the Commission on the Future of Health and Social Care in England, 2014, Wenzel et al, 2018 and the House of Lords, 2019). Significantly, the government has gone down the hypothecated route with its new health and social care levy from 2023. Alternatively, it could have adopted the Japanese approach of requiring a specific contribution from the over-40s, recognising that they will benefit the most from better long-term care.

Considering taxation of wealth as a future funding source: the UK tax system is heavily skewed towards raising revenue from employment rather than wealth and capital. One of the major social changes since 1948 noted in Chapter 2 has been the unprecedented levels of household wealth. This is distributed twice as unequally as income and much of it is concentrated in older age groups who will benefit the most from higher spending on social care (Advani et al, 2020). House price growth alone over the past 20 years has delivered an 'unearned, unequal and untaxed £3 trillion capital gains windfall, with those aged 60 and over the biggest winners' (Corlett and Leslie, 2021). So, there is a persuasive argument for funding some of this through taxation of wealth, including property. The LSE Wealth Commission has argued that any future tax rises in response to COVID-19 should take the form of a one-off wealth tax in preference to increasing taxes on work or spending. It estimates that a one-off wealth tax on millionaire couples paid at 1 per cent a year for five years would raise £260 billion (Advani et al, 2021). Alternative options include changes to existing taxes – inheritance tax, capital gains tax and/or council tax.

A long-term approach to funding reform will be necessary. The likely quantum of money needed to implement a new social contract and changes to the design and delivery of social care put forward earlier will not be raised in one fell swoop. Rather, it will be a staged process over many years that can be adjusted to changing fortunes of the economy. A multi-year financial settlement akin to, and ideally in parallel with, the NHS settlement will be needed. This would make it easier for councils and care providers to plan together over a longer period instead of being constrained by short-term injections of money. Ideally, the settlement should be informed by regular forecasts of needs and funding requirements, conducted independently of central government. This could be a role for the Office of Budget Responsibility and linked to the national spending review process. Establishing a long-term funding settlement will help the state become as much a smart spender as a high spender.

Private funding will remain a significant funding source for years to come, given the scale of private wealth and the certainty that people should wish to draw on this to live a better life in their later years. But it cannot be right that those with a degree of wealth, even of modest proportions, face the prospect of worse outcomes as a result of distress purchases and poor, uninformed choices. In a pluralistic democracy, the boundaries of social care should extend beyond municipalism. Instead of seeing self-funders as entirely separate from the public system of care, the state's role could be to help people plan ahead, using their own resources, through better advice and support from the new independent advisory centres proposed earlier. The introduction of the cap on care costs from 2023, if it goes ahead, will help by gradually bringing self-funders on to the radar of councils.

Alongside an adequately funded and well-designed system of public funding, more could be done to enable private wealth to complement public provision. People can be encouraged to see planning for future care needs in the same way as planning for future housing or pension needs; to have choices not simply about protecting their savings and assets, but how they can use their resources to have a better quality of life. Ideas include immediate needs annuities, care ISAs, equity release and pension and other tax reliefs against spending on care (Adams, 2019).

There needs to be changes to the governance of social care funding. The current funding flows within social care are of byzantine complexity, involving at least seven separate funding sources and little transparency or accountability. This results in a cycle of mutual blame between central government, councils and care providers. This muddle has made it all too easy for the government to hide behind a cloak of confusion and, over many years, shift the costs of care onto the shoulders of individuals, families and council-tax-payers, while at the same time maintaining it has given councils all they need to pay for local services.

Instead, discussions about a new funding settlement could examine the possibility of moving towards some kind of capitation funding or national fee rates for local care services. These could be set nationally by central government but take account of differences in cost in different places. There are plenty of precedents, such as the national funding formula through which the government funds individual schools and the national system of NHS tariff payments for hospital and other services. Australia has established an Independent Pricing Authority to set fee levels, and other countries with social insurance schemes have similar vehicles to determine payments to care providers. At a stroke, the government would then, for the first time, have 'skin in the game' by requiring them to take responsibility for the direct consequences of their funding decisions and what local services receive. It would also detoxify the difficult relationships in some places between councils and providers and enable them to focus on the local planning of services. Collaborative relationships about innovation and planning would replace adversarial conflicts about fee levels. Moving towards a stronger national funding regime would, however, represent a major upheaval in the financial wiring of the social care system. It would be time-consuming and far from straightforward, and a through appraisal of the pros and cons would be essential.

Agreeing a new funding settlement for social care calls for another change, at national level, concerning the role of HM Treasury; a change which is perhaps less about governance per se and more about culture and attitudes. The traditional role of the Treasury has been to act as the custodian of the public purse, with a congenital disposition to resist any calls for new spending. For social care, this has been a profound obstacle to reform because the Treasury knows that the costs of care can be surreptitiously directed away from the public purse towards self-funders, council-tax-payers and the NHS (Figure 3.2). As Anita Charlesworth and her colleagues have pointed out, however, the role of the Treasury is not just to look at costs but to be a guardian of the country's economic wellbeing, overseeing how well markets work for people and how public spending can benefit individuals and society as a whole (Charlesworth et al, 2021). The Treasury's thinking and decision-making about social care should be driven less by the costs to the Exchequer and more by its contribution to the economic and social infrastructure of the country.

Conclusion

The Johnson government's proposals, while not without merit, fall well short of the scale of change and ambition that is necessary to resolve one of the most pressing domestic policy challenges the country faces. They do not offer a plan that will 'fix the crisis in social care once and for all.' That will not be achieved by tinkering with the existing system and leaving the growing human and financial costs of failure to rest even more heavily on the shoulders of individuals and families or an underpaid and undervalued workforce. Nor will it be achieved by invoking a hazily defined concept of a national care service that overlooks the fact that social care is fundamentally different from health care and ignores the dismal track record of the NHS in providing non-curative care.

Instead, this book sets out a prospectus for long term reform through:

- a new social contract for care that sets out the mutual roles and responsibilities of individuals, families, communities and the state (at national and local levels) – a contract based on the simple idea that most of us will give and receive support at some point in our lives;
- a different model of design and delivery that gives people new rights and resources to shape the care and support arrangements that work for them and offers peace of mind to everyone who needs care now or will do so in the future;
- a new funding settlement that positions social care as a major, universal public service in its own right, finally dispersing the shadows cast by the Victorian Poor Law and the post-war welfare state from which social care was missing. This should rest on a view that any advanced economy depends on good social care as part of the economic

and social infrastructure in the same way that it depends on investments in education, skills and health care.

To achieve these profound changes will be difficult and take time. It will depend on a fundamentally different approach to policy-making that seeks to build sufficient support for change by engaging directly with the public through participatory democracy and with people who have care and support needs, through co-production. It entails rejecting short-term-initiativitis for a sustainable, long-term approach and learning from the past instead of repeating it. The prize will be a modern social care system characterised not by factories of care dependency, but by a range of supports and services that enable people to lead the best lives they can, whatever their needs or circumstances, and participate as valued citizens in society.

The American campaigner Ai–jen Poo offers a pithy reminder of why care has become such an important and universal feature of all our lives. Care, she says, is:

> The most fundamental form of support that we offer others that we love and know in our lives. And it's something we rely on from the time that we're born to the time that we take our last breath. All of us need and rely on care and provide it at different points in our lives. And so that's why we say it's essential. It's the work that makes all other work possible. (New York Times, 2021)

In 1942, John Maynard Keynes argued for the reconstruction of the nation's economic and social infrastructure after the devastation of war with the words, 'Assuredly we can afford this and so much more. Anything we can actually do, we can afford.' When the welfare state was constructed amid the ruins of the Second World War, the national debt stood at 251 per cent of GDP. Today, that figure is 82 per cent (ONS, 2021d). In the century of COVID-19, surely it is a matter of not whether the country can afford better social care, but how can it afford not to.

Postscript

Tumultuous political and economic developments have unfolded since this book was submitted for publication.

In Boris Johnson's final speech as Prime Minister outside Downing Street in September 2022, he included social care in a list of manifesto commitments he professed to be 'proud' to have delivered, a claim at odds with accumulating evidence that social care remains far from fixed. As an issue it was barely raised at all during the leadership debates that preceded the appointment of Liz Truss as his successor, although she did pledge her intention to reverse the National Insurance rise introduced in April to provide more money for health and social care, with it to be raised through higher taxation instead. She argued, to the consternation of NHS leaders, that social care should get a bigger share of the proceeds because the NHS has already received "quite a lot". An expected emergency Budget in the autumn will no doubt clarify whether robbing Peter to pay Paul is the new administration's strategy to funding health and social care.

Although most elements of the government's limited funding reforms show no sign of being abandoned, alarm bells have begun to ring. The Local Government Association has called for delay, arguing as it did in 2015 that the changes need more time and more money. It remains to be seen whether the reforms will unravel, with history again repeating itself. Even if they proceed, the new political mood music favouring a smaller state, lower taxes and de-regulation does not encourage optimism about the appetite of the Truss Government for further action to address the deeper problems in social care laid out in this book. Much may depend on the views of the new Secretary of State for Health and Social Care, the third postholder in as many months, the twelfth in twenty-five years. The absence of long-term continuity in national political leadership and policy direction has never been more apparent.

In the meantime, having barely recovered from the shock of COVID-19, the economic environment has deteriorated sharply since Russia's invasion of Ukraine, with catastrophic rises in energy prices, record levels of inflation, rising interest rates and the economy on the edge of recession. This has profound consequences for private households and public finances. We are set to become a poorer country. The Institute for Fiscal Studies estimates that 40 per cent of the extra money the government was planning to put into public services, including the NHS and social care, will be wiped out by higher inflation. Signs from across the Atlantic are no more encouraging. President Biden received much acclaim for securing legislation to tackle climate change and reduce health care and energy costs – the oddly-named Inflation Reduction Act – but at the cost of abandoning the bold plans in the original 'Build Back Better' proposals to invest substantially in home and family care.

In this vortex of policy uncertainty, economic challenge and competing domestic and international crises, arguing the case for investment and reform in adult social care has become even harder. The imperative of managing and reacting to immediate crises is likely once again to perpetuate a focus on short-term fixes at the expense of seeking sustainable long-term solutions. The deepening summer crisis in NHS emergency care highlights its essential inter-dependency with social care and the heavy price now being paid for a decade and more of policy neglect, under-investment and short-term thinking. But we should not allow the dreadful economic and fiscal climate to extinguish hope that fundamental change is possible, as the post-war Welfare State testifies. If anything, recent events strengthen the case for social care investment as an integral feature of economic and social reconstruction and recovery. That spending choices are a matter of relative priorities, not whether they are affordable in an absolute sense, has been demonstrated again by the speed of the Truss government's willingness to find at least £100 billion of new money – more than four times current annual public spending on social care – to protect people from soaring energy prices. While the new road to reform proposed in this book has become much steeper, its importance to the quality of our lives is as great as ever. Care remains, in the words of Ai-jen Poo, 'The work that makes all other work possible'.[1]

Notes

Chapter 2
[1] Commonly referred to as 'bed blocking' a term rejected here as it implies it is the patient's fault for occupying the bed, whereas it is the poor operation of the system that is blocking the patient's discharge.

Chapter 3
[1] The questions asked were, 'How satisfied or dissatisfied are you with social care provided by local authorities for people who cannot look after themselves because of illness, disability or old age?' and 'In the past 12 months ... have you used or had contact with any of the following services? This could be for yourself or someone else?'

Chapter 4
[1] https://everyaustraliancounts.com.au/about
[2] https://caringacross.org/why-care/

Chapter 7
[1] Co-production has been defined as 'when you as an individual influence the support and services you receive, or when groups of people get together to influence the way that services are designed, commissioned and delivered' (DHSC, 2021a).
[2] https://engagebritain.org/challenge/health-care

Postscript
[1] https://www.ted.com/talks/ai_jen_poo_the_work_that_makes_all_other_work_possible

References

Abel-Smith, B. and Townsend, P. (1965) The Poor and the Poorest: A New Analysis of the Ministry of Labour's Family Expenditure Surveys of 1953–54 and 1960, London: Bell & Sons.

Adam, S., Hodge, L., Phillips, D. and Xu, X. (2020) Revaluation and reform: Bringing council tax into the 21st century, London: Institute of Fiscal Studies, Available from: https://www.ifs.org.uk/uploads/R168-Revaluation-and-reform-bringing-council-tax-in-England-into-the-21st-century-updated.pdf [Accessed 19 January 2022].

Adams, J. (2019) Care in later life: incentives to use assets to pay for care, Pensions Policy Institute Research Paper, Available from: https://www.pensionspolicyinstitute.org.uk/media/3212/20190625-care-in-later-life-incentives-to-use-assets-to-pay-for-care.pdf [Accessed 21 December 2021].

Advani, A., Bangham, G. and Leslie, J. (2020) The UK's wealth distribution and characteristics of high-wealth households, Resolution Foundation, Available from: https://www.resolutionfoundation.org/app/uploads/2020/12/The-UKs-wealth-distribution.pdf [Accessed 20 December 2021].

Advani, A., Chamberlain, E. and Summers, A. (2021) Wealth Tax for the UK: Wealth Tax Commission Final Report, Available from: https://www.wealthandpolicy.com/wp/WealthTaxFinalReport.pdf [Accessed 20 December 2021].

Andrew, A., Bandiera, O., Costa-Dias, M. and Landais, C. (2021) Women and Men from Work, IFS Deaton Review of Inequalities, Available from: https://ifs.org.uk/inequality/women-and-men-at-work [Accessed 7 December 2021].

Appleby, J. (2016) Is the UK spending more than we thought on healthcare (and much less on social care)? Data Briefing, British Medical Journal, Available from: https://doi.org/10.1136/bmj.i3094 [Accessed 16 January 2022].

Appleby, J., Hemmings, N., Maguire, D., Morris, J., Schlepper, L. and Wellings, D. (2020) Public Satisfaction with the NHS and Social Care in 2019: Results and Trends from the British Social Attitudes Survey, Research Report, Nuffield Trust and The King's Fund, Available from: https://www.kingsfund.org.uk/publications/public-satisfaction-nhs-social-care-2019#introduction https://www.kingsfund.org.uk/publications/public-satisfaction-nhs-social-care-2019#social-care [Accessed 16 January 2022].

Association of British Insurers (2014) Developing products for social care, Available from: http://www.abi.org.uk/globalassets/sitecore/files/documents/publications/public/2014/social-care/developing-products-for-social-care-report.pdf [Accessed 16 January 2022].

Association of Directors of Social Services (ADASS) (2015) Distinctive, valued, personal: Why adult social care matters – the next five years.

ADASS (2020) Autumn Survey 2020, Available from: https://www.adass.org.uk/media/8305/adass-autumn-survey-report-2020_final-website.pdf [Accessed 16 January 2022].

ADASS (2021) Spring Survey, Available from: https://www.adass.org.uk/media/8766/adass-spring-survey-report-2021-final-no-embargo.pdf [Accessed 16 January 2022].

ADASS (2021a) Home Care and Workforce Snap Survey September 2021, Available from: https://www.adass.org.uk/media/8984/final-rapid-survey-report-070921-publication-updated.docx [Accessed 16 January 2022].

ADASS (2021b) Home Care and Workforce Rapid Survey November 2021, Available from: https://www.adass.org.uk/media/8987/adass-snap-survey-report-november-2021.pdf [Accessed 28 November 2021].

Archbishop of Canterbury (2021) Archbishop's Commission Reimagining Care, Available from: https://www.archbishopofcanterbury.org/priorities/archbishops-commission-reimagining-care/about-reimagining-care-commission [Accessed 16 January 2022].

Astor, M. (2019) How the politically unthinkable can become mainstream, New York Times [online] 26 February, Available from: https://www.nytimes.com/2019/02/26/us/politics/overton-window-democrats.html [Accessed 16 January 2022].

Attlee, C. (1920) The Social Worker, London: G. Bell.

Australian Government (2012) Living longer, living better: Aged care reform package, Available from: https://www.health.gov.au/sites/default/files/documents/2019/10/foi-request-1295-extra-service-fees-living-longer-living-better-aged-care-reform-package-april-2012_0.pdf [Accessed 16 January 2022].

Australian Government (2021) Schedule of fees and charges for residential and home care: From 1 July 2021, Department of Health, Available from: https://www.health.gov.au/sites/default/documents/2021/06/schedule-of-fees-and-charges-for-residential-and-home-care-schedule-from-1-july-2021_0.pdf [Accessed 16 January 2022].

Australian Government (2021a) Australian Government Response to the Final Report of the Royal Commission into Aged Care Quality and Safety, Available from: https://www.health.gov.au/sites/default/files/documents/2021/05/australian-government-response-to-the-final-report-of-the-royal-commission-into-aged-care-quality-and-safety.pdf [Accessed 16 January 2022].

Australian Institute of Health and Welfare (2018) Older Australia from a Glance, Web Report, Available from: https://www.aihw.gov.au/reports/older-people/older-australia-at-a-glance/contents/health-aged-care-service-use/aged-care-assessments [Accessed 16 January 2022].

Bambra, B., Lynch, J. and Smith, K. (2021) The Unequal Pandemic COVID-19 and Health Inequalities, Bristol: Policy Press.

Bangham, G. and Leslie, L. (2020) Rainy days: An audit of household wealth and the initial effects of the coronavirus crisis on saving and spending in Great Britain, Available from: https://www.resolutionfoundation.org/app/uploads/2020/06/Rainy-Days.pdf [Accessed 18 January 2022].

Barclay, P. (1982) Social Workers: Their Role and Tasks, London: National Institute for Social Work.

BBC (2017) Today, 18 May 2017, Available from: https://www.bbc.co.uk/programmes/b08q317m [Accessed 11 January 2022].

BBC (2019) Reflections, 12 August, Available from: https://www.bbc.co.uk/programmes/m0007k5h [Accessed 4 January 2022].

BBC News (2013) Andrew Dilnot: Social care cap higher than we wanted, 1 February, Available from: https://www.bbc.co.uk/news/av/health-21408949 [Accessed 15 January 2022].

BBC News (2017) General election: Theresa May denies social care U-turn, 22 May, Available from: https://www.bbc.co.uk/news/election-2017-40001221 [Accessed December 17 2021].

BBC News (2020) Coronavirus: Isle of Wight care workers live in tents, 23 April, Available from: https://www.bbc.co.uk/news/av/uk-england-hampshire-52379392 [Accessed October 24 2021].

BBC News (2021) Help: Channel 4 drama examines 'undervalued' care workers during pandemic, 16 September, Available from: https://www.bbc.co.uk/news/entertainment-arts-58537568 [Accessed 20 October 2021].

BBC News (2021a) Amazon offers £1,000 joining bonus for new UK staff website, 24 August, Available from: https://www.bbc.co.uk/news/business-58321728 [Accessed November 2 2021].

BBC News (2021b) 100 people held more than 20 years in 'institutions', 24 November, Available from: https://www.bbc.co.uk/news/uk-59388886 [Accessed 2 January 2022].

Bennett, A. (2008) Untold Stories, London: Faber & Faber.

Bennett, L. and Humphries, R. (2014) Making best use of the Better Care Fund: Spending to save? London: The King's Fund, Available from: https://www.kingsfund.org.uk/publications/making-best-use-better-care-fund [Accessed 18 January 2022].

Bentley, D. (2010) Parties' row over care reform grows, The Independent, 15 February, Available from: https://www.independent.co.uk/news/uk/politics/parties-row-over-care-reform-grows-1899542.html [Accessed 10 August 2021].

Blair, T. (1997) Leader's speech, Brighton, British Political Speech, Available from: http://www.britishpoliticalspeech.org/speech-archive.htm?speech=203 [Accessed 4 July 2021].

Blake, D. and Orszag M. (1999) Annual estimates of personal wealth holdings in the United Kingdom since 1948, Applied Financial Economics, 9:4, 397–421.

Bogdanor, V. (1999) Devolution in the United Kingdom, Oxford: Oxford University Press.

Bolton, J. (2016) Predicting and managing demand in adult social care, Oxford: Institute of Public Care, Available from: https://ipc.brookes.ac.uk/docs/John_Bolton_Predicting_and_managing_demand_in_social_care-IPC_discussion_paper_April_2016.pdf [Accessed 14 January 2022].

Bosch, I. (2021) Under pressure: NHS priorities this winter, NHS Confederation, Available from: https://www.nhsconfed.org/publications/under-pressure [Accessed 14 December 2021].

Bottery, S. (2019) What's your problem, social care? The eight key areas for reform, Available from: https://www.kingsfund.org.uk/publications/whats-your-problem-social-care# [Accessed 14 January 2022].

Bottery, S. and Ward, D. (2021) Social Care 360, London: The King's Fund.

Brindle, D. (2008) Registering disapproval, The Guardian [online] 2 July https://www.theguardian.com/society/2008/jul/02/longtermcare.socialcare1 [Accessed 14 January 2022].

British Geriatrics Society (2021) Right time, right place: Urgent community-based care for older people, Available from: https://www.bgs.org.uk/righttimerightplace [Accessed 18 December 2021].

Brown, G. (2017) My Life, Our Times, London: Vintage

Buck, D., Baylis A., Dougall, D. and Robinson, R. (2018) A vision for population health: Towards a healthier future, London: The King's Fund, Available from: https://www.kingsfund.org.uk/sites/default/files/2018-11/A%20vision%20for%20population%20health%20online%20version.pdf [Accessed 6 December 2021].

Bunting, M. (2020) Labours of Love: The Crisis of Care, London: Granta.

Burchardt, T. (2020) Does COVID-19 represent a 'new Beveridge' moment, a crisis that will wash away, or a call to action? Report of a roundtable discussion on theories of welfare, LSE Centre for Analysis of Social Exclusion, Available from: https://sticerd.lse.ac.uk/dps/case/spdo/spdorn02.pdf [Accessed 14 January 2022].

Butler, P. (2021) At least 75,000 people in England wait six months for social care assessment, The Guardian, 14 July, Available from: https://www.theguardian.com/society/2021/jul/14/adult-social-care-waiting-lists-in-england-condemned-as-unacceptable [Accessed 14 January 2022].

Butler, P. and Saper, E. (2021) Fixing Social Care: New funding, New Methods, New Partnerships, London: Adam Smith Institute.

Buzelli, L., Cameron, G. and Gardner, T. (2022) Public perceptions of the NHS and social care: Performance, policy and expectations, Health Foundation, Available from: https://www.health.org.uk/publications/long-reads/public-perceptions-performance-policy-and-expectations [Accessed 14 February 2022].

Cabinet Office (2010) The Coalition: Our programme for government, Available from: https://assets.publishing.service.gov.uk/government/uploads/system/uploads/attachment_data/file/78977/coalition_programme_for_government.pdf [Accessed 14 January 2022].

Cameron, D. (2019) For the Record, London: William Collins.

Campbell, J. (2006) Opinion: Registration should be a matter of choice, Available from: https://www.communitycare.co.uk/2006/11/02/opinion-registration-should-be-a-matter-of-choice/ [Accessed 14 January 2022].

Care and Support Alliance (2015) CSA responds to care cap deferral, Available from http://careandsupportalliance.com/csa-welcomes-care-cap-deferral/ [Accessed 7 December 2021].

Care and Support Alliance (2021) CSA's statement in response to the White Paper on social care, 1 December 1, Available from: https://careandsupportalliance.com/csas-statement-in-response-to-the-white-paper-on-social-care/ [Accessed 31 December 2021].

Care England (2021) 1948 moment for social care, Available from: https://www.careengland.org.uk/news/1948-moment-adult-social-care [Accessed 14 January 2022].

Care Quality Commission (2021) The state of health care and adult social care in England 2020/21, HC 753, Available from: https://www.cqc.org.uk/sites/default/files/20211021_stateofcare2021_print.pdf [Accessed 15 December 2022].

Care Quality Commission (2022) Appendix A to Executive Team Report to the Board (Chief Inspector of Adult Social Care's report): Update on adult social care workforce [online], 23 February, Available from: https://www.cqc.org.uk/sites/default/files/20220221_ET_Update_Appendix_Feb-22_ASC_workforce_WEB.docx [Accessed 25 February 2022].

Carers UK (2020) Unseen and undervalued: the value of unpaid care provided to date during the COVID-19 pandemic, Report, Available from: https://www.carersuk.org/for-professionals/policy/policy-library/unseen-and-undervalued-the-value-of-unpaid-care-provided-to-date-during-the-COVID-19-pandemic [Accessed 11 November 2021].

Carers UK (2020a) Carer's Week 2020 Research Report: The Rise in the Number of Unpaid Carers During the Coronavirus (COVID-19) Outbreak, London: Carers UK.

Caring Across Generations (2021) Long-term care in Build Back Better garners broad support, [blog] 14 September, https://caringacross.org/blog/blog-build-back-better-broad-support/ [Accessed 14 January 2022].

Caring Choices (2008) The future of care: Funding time for a change, London, The King's Fund, Available from: https://www.kingsfund.org.uk/sites/default/files/future-of-care-funding-time-change-caring-choices-kings-fund-january-2008.pdf [Accessed 14 January 2022].

Carter, C. (2021) Social care cuts and increased charges causing 'huge distress' to disabled people, Community Care, 13 April, Available from: https://www.communitycare.co.uk/2021/04/13/social-care-cuts-increased-charges-causing-huge-distress-disabled-people/ [Accessed 14 January 2022].

Castle, S. (2020) 'The new Church of England': Coronavirus renews pride in UK's health service, New York Times, 12 May, Available from: https://www.nytimes.com/2020/05/12/world/europe/coronavirus-nhs-uk.html [Accessed 14 January 2022].

Cavendish, C. (2019) Extra Time: Ten Lessons for an Ageing World, London: Harper Collins.

Cecil, N. (2019) Brexit has delayed plans to deal with adult social care crisis, minister admits, Evening Standard, 12 February, Available from: https://www.standard.co.uk/news/politics/brexit-has-delayed-plans-to-deal-with-adult-social-care-crisis-minister-admits-a4064436.html [Accessed 14 January 2022].

Centre for Ageing Better (2020) An old age problem? How society shapes and reinforces negative attitudes to ageing, report, Available from: https://www.ageing-better.org.uk/sites/default/files/2020-11/old-age-problem.pdf [Accessed 14 January 2022].

Chambers, D., Cantrell, A. and Booth, A. (2019) Rapid evidence review: why do people enter the adult social care workforce in the UK and why do they leave? University of Sheffield School of Health and Related Research.

Charles, A. (2021) Integrated care systems explained: making sense of systems, places and neighbourhoods, The King's Fund, Available from: https://www.kingsfund.org.uk/publications/integrated-care-systems-explained [Accessed 12 August 2021].

Charlesworth, A., Tallack, C. and Alderwick, H. (2021) If not now, when? The long overdue promise of social care reform, Available from: https://www.health.org.uk/news-and-comment/blogs/if-not-now-when-the-long-overdue-promise-of-social-care-reform [Accessed 4 November 2021].

CICTAR (2021) Death, deception and dividends, Available from: https://cictar.org/wp-content/uploads/2021/12/Death-Deception-Dividends-Dec-3.5.pdf [Accessed 15 December 2021].

Coats, D. (2020) A new Beveridge, Fabian Society, Available from: https://fabians.org.uk/a-new-beveridge/ [Accessed 6 December 2021].

Cohn, D. (2021) Why a transformation of caregiving could be Biden's BFD, Huffpost, 19 September, Available from: https://www.huffingtonpost.co.uk/entry/biden-democratic-child-care-paid-leave-hcbs-agenda_n_61457709e4b0efa77f80410a [Accessed January 6 2022].

Comas-Herrera, A., Butterfield, R., Fernández, J.L. and Wittenberg, R. (2012) Barriers to and opportunities for private long-term care insurance in England: What can we learn from other countries? in McGuire, A. and Costa-Font, J. (eds), LSE Companion to Health Policy, Cheltenham: Edward Elgar.

Commission on the Future of Health and Social Care in England (2014) A new settlement for health and social care, interim report, London: The King's Fund, Available from: https://www.kingsfund.org.uk/publications/new-settlement-health-and-social-care-interim [Accessed 8 December 2021].

Commission on the Future of Health and Social Care in England (2014a) A new settlement for health and social care, Final Report, London: The King's Fund, Available from: https://www.kingsfund.org.uk/publications/new-settlement-health-and-social-care [Accessed 8 December 2021].

Competition and Markets Authority (2017) Care homes market study final report, Available from: https://assets.publishing.service.gov.uk/media/5a1fdf30e5274a750b82533a/care-homes-market-study-final-report.pdf [Accessed 14 January 2021].

Congressional Budget Office (2021) Economic effects of expanding home- and community-based services in Medicaid, Available from: https://www.cbo.gov/system/files/2021-11/57632-Medicaid.pdf [Accessed 28 November 2021].

Conservative and Unionist Party (2017) Forward together: Our plan for a stronger Britain and a prosperous future, The Conservative and Unionist Party Manifesto 2017. London: Conservative and Unionist Party.

Corlett, A. and Leslie, J. (2021) Home county options for taxing main residence capital gains, briefing note, London: Resolution Foundation, Available from: https://www.resolutionfoundation.org/app/uploads/2021/12/Home-county.pdf [Accessed 17 January 2022].

County Council Network and Newton (2021) The future of adult social care, Available from: https://www.futureasc.com/ [Accessed 12 December 2021].

Cozens, A. (2003) Taking down the fences: Redefining social services in local government presidential address, Association of Directors of Social Services, October 2003, unpublished.

Craig, J. (2021) A healthy living: Four stories from the future of care, Available from: https://www.carecity.london/publications/reports/33-healthy-living-four-stories-from-the-future-of-care/file [Accessed 22 December 2022].

Crawford, R., Stoye G. and Zaranko, B. (2021) Long-term care spending and hospital use among the older population in England, Journal of Health Economics, Volume 78, July 2021, 102477, Available from: https://doi.org/10.1016/j.jhealeco.2021.102477 [Accessed 17 January 2022].

Crowther, N. (2020) A long-term framework to transform social care?, Social Care Future, blog post, 1 December, Available from: https://socialcarefuture.blog/2020/12/01/a-long-term-framework-for-changing-social-care/ [Accessed 17 January 2022].

Crowther, N. (2021) Want to help change the story of social care? Follow these basic rules, Social Care Future, blog post, 20 April, Available from: https://socialcarefuture.blog/2021/04/20/want-to-help-change-the-story-of-social-care-follow-these-basic-rules/ [Accessed 17 January 2022].

Crowther, N. and Quinton, K. (2021) How to build public support to transform social care: A practical guide for communicating about social care, Report, Available from: https://socialcarefuture.blog/how-to-build-public-support-to-transform-social-care-a-practical-guide/ [Accessed 17 January 2022].

Curry, N. (2017) Looking to the long term: The Japanese approach, Nuffield Trust, Available from: https://www.nuffieldtrust.org. uk/news-item/looking-to-the-long-term-the-japanese-approach [Accessed 17 January 2022].

Curry, N., Castle-Clarke, S. and Hemmings, N. (2018) What can England learn from the long-term care system in Japan? Research Report, London: Nuffield Trust, Available from: https://www. nuffieldtrust.org.uk/research/what-can-england-learn-from-the-long-term-care-system-in-japan#lessons-for-england [Accessed 5 August 2020].

Curry, N., Schlepper, L. and Hemmings, N. (2019) What can England learn from the long-term care system in Germany? Research Report, London: Nuffield Trust, Available from: https://www.nuffieldtr ust.org.uk/research/what-can-england-learn-from-the-long-term-care-system-in-germany#what-next-for-england [Accessed 17 January 2022].

Cylus, J., Roland, D., Nolte, E., Corbett, J., Jones, K., Forder, J. and Sussex, J. (2018) Identifying options for funding the NHS and social care in the UK: International evidence, London: Health Foundation.

D'Arcy, C. and Gardiner, L. (2017) The generation of wealth: Asset accumulation across and within cohorts, London: Resolution Foundation, Available from: https://www.resolutionfoundation. org/publications/the-generation-of-wealth-asset-accumulation-acr oss-and-within-cohorts/ [Accessed 28 December 2021].

Davey, V. (2020) Regulation of care workers: Should personal assistants be included? Blog, Think Local Act Personal, 26 February, Available from: https://www.thinklocalactpersonal.org.uk/Blog/Regulation-of-care-workers-should-personal-assistants-be-included/ [Accessed 17 January 2022].

Davies, N., Campbell, C. and McNulty, C. (2018) How to fix the funding of health and social care, Report, London: Institute of Government, Available from: https://www.instituteforgovernm ent.org.uk/publications/how-fix-funding-health-and-social-care [Accessed 17 January 2022].

Davy, L. (2019) So you're thinking of going into a nursing home? Here's what you'll have to pay for, UNSW, 16 May, Available from: https://newsroom.unsw.edu.au/news/social-affairs/so-youre-thinking-going-nursing-home-heres-what-youll-have-pay [Accessed 17 November 2021].

Department of Health (1989) Caring for people: Community care in the next decade and beyond, Cm 849, London: HMSO.

Department of Health (1998) Modernising social services: Promoting independence, improving protection, Raising standards, Cm 4169, London: HMSO, Available from: https://webarchive.nationalarchives. gov.uk/20131205101158/http://www.archive.official-documents. co.uk/document/cm41/4169/4169.htm [Accessed 17 January 2022].

Department of Health (2005) Independence, well-being and choice, Cm 6499, London: HMSO.

Department of Health (2010) Vision for adult social care: Capable communities and active citizens, London: Department of Health, Available from: https://webarchive.nationalarchives.gov.uk/2012110 7104731/http://www.dh.gov.uk/prod_consum_dh/groups/dh_di gitalassets/@dh/@en/@ps/documents/digitalasset/dh_121971.pdf [Accessed 17 January 2022].

Department of Health (2012) Long term conditions compendium of information: Third edition, London: Department of Health, Available from: https://assets.publishing.service.gov.uk/government/uplo ads/system/uploads/attachment_data/file/216528/dh_134486.pdf [Accessed 17 January 2022].

Department of Health (2013) The Cavendish Review: An independent review into healthcare assistants and support workers in the NHS and social care settings, Available from: https://assets.publishing.service. gov.uk/government/uploads/system/uploads/attachment_data/file/ 236212/Cavendish_Review.pdf [Accessed 17 January 2022].

Department of Health (2015) Delay in the implementation of the cap care costs, Correspondence, Available from: https://www.gov.uk/gov ernment/publications/delay-in-the-implementation-of-the-cap-on-care-costs [Accessed 17 January 2022].

DHSC (Department of Health and Social Care) (2020) Health and Social Care Secretary's statement on coronavirus (COVID-19), 15 April, Available from: https://www.gov.uk/government/speeches/ health-and-social-care-secretarys-statement-on-coronavirus-covid-19-15-april-2020 [Accessed 17 January 2022].

DHSC (2020a) Social Care Sector: COVID-19 Support Taskforce full recommendations including all Advisory Group recommendations, Available from: https://assets.publishing.service.gov.uk/government/uploads/system/uploads/attachment_data/file/919113/20200917_Taskforce_report_recommendations_FINAL.pdf [Accessed 5 August 2021).

DHSC (2020b) Better Care Fund: policy statement 2020 to 2021, London: Department of Health and Social Care, Available from: https://www.gov.uk/government/publications/better-care-fund-policy-statement-2020-to-2021/better-care-fund-policy-statement-2020-to-2021#better-care-fund-2020-to-2021 [Accessed 17 January 2022].

DHSC (2021) Statement of impact: The Health and Social Care Act 2008 (Regulated Activities) (Amendment) (Coronavirus) Regulations 2021, Available from: https://www.gov.uk/government/consultations/making-vaccination-a-condition-of-deployment-in-older-adult-care-homes/outcome/statement-of-impact-the-health-and-social-care-act-2008-regulated-activities-amendment-coronavirus-regulations-2021 [Accessed on 17 January 2022].

DHSC (2021a) Evidence review for Adult Social Care Reform, Available from: https://assets.publishing.service.gov.uk/government/uploads/system/uploads/attachment_data/file/1037884/evidence-review-for-adult-social-care-reform.pdf [Accessed on 7 January 2022].

DHSC (2021b) Policy paper Adult social care: COVID-19 winter plan 2021 to 2022; Workforce Capacity Fund for adult social care; Workforce Recruitment and Retention Fund for adult social care; Adult social care campaign to build bigger and better workforce, 3 November, Available from: https://www.gov.uk/government/publications/workforce-capacity-fund-for-adult-social-care [Accessed 17 January 2022].

DHSC (2021c) People at the heart of care: Adult social care reform, White Paper, CP 560, London: HMSO.

DHSC (2021d) Impact statement: Making vaccination a condition of deployment in health and wider social care sector, Available from: https://assets.publishing.service.gov.uk/government/uploads/system/uploads/attachment_data/file/1032255/making-vaccination-a-condition-of-deployment-in-the-health-and-wider-social-care-sector-impact_statement.pdf [Accessed 28 November 2021].

DHSC (2021e) Biggest visa boost for social care as Health and Care Visa scheme expanded, Press Release, 24 December, Available from: https://www.gov.uk/government/news/biggest-visa-boost-for-social-care-as-health-and-care-visa-scheme-expanded [Accessed 29 December 2021].

DHSC (2022) Care and support statutory guidance, Available from: https://www.gov.uk/government/publications/care-act-statut ory-guidance/care-and-support-statutory-guidance [Accessed 31 May 2022].

DHSC (2022a) Impact statement: Adult Social Care System Reform statement of impact for the white paper, 'People at the heart of care: adult social care reform' (December 2021), Available from: https://assets.publishing.service.gov.uk/government/uploads/ system/uploads/attachment_data/file/1056192/adult_social_care_sys tem_reform_impact_statement.pdf [Accessed 5 April 2022].

DHSC (2022b) 'Made with Care' website, Available from: https:// www.adultsocialcare.co.uk/home.aspx [Accessed 18 May 2022].

Department of Work and Pensions (2020) Benefit expenditure and caseload tables 2020, Available from: https://www.gov.uk/governm ent/publications/benefit-expenditure-and-caseload-tables-2020 [Accessed 17 January 2022].

Department of Work and Pensions (2021) Shaping future support: The health and disability green paper, CP470, London: HMSO, Available from: https://assets.publishing.service.gov.uk/government/ uploads/system/uploads/attachment_data/file/1004042/shaping-fut ure-support-the-health-and-disability-green-paper.pdf [Accessed 17 January 2022].

Dilnot Report (2011) Fairer care funding: The report of the Commission on Funding of Care and Support, Available from: https://webarchive. nationalarchives.gov.uk/20120713201059/http://www.dilnotcom mission.dh.gov.uk/files/2011/07/Fairer-Care-Funding-Report.pdf [Accessed 17 January 2022].

Dixon, A. (2020) The Age of Ageing Better? A Manifesto for our Future, London: Green Tree.

Dunn, P., Allen, L., Alarilla, A., Grimm, F., Humphries, R. and Alderwick, H. (2021) Adult social care and COVID-19 after the first wave: Assessing the policy response in England – Our analysis of the national government policy response for social care between June 2020 and March 2021, London: Health Foundation.

Elliott, F. (2021) Careless whispers: A short history of social care reform and why the conversation needs to change to avoid more failure, London: Engage Britain, Available from: https://engagebritain.org/wp-content/uploads/Careless-Whispers-Engage-Britain-Final.pdf [Accessed 17 January 2022].

Elliott, F., Coates, S. and Jones, C. (2018) Theresa May ditches key pledges to prepare for no-deal Brexit: Social care reform threatened by Brexit turmoil The Times, 19 December, Available from: https://www.thetimes.co.uk/article/theresa-may-ditches-key-pledges-to-prepare-for-no-deal-brexit-0rqfl7f7x [Accessed 17 January 2022].

Elstub, S. and Carrick, J. (2019) Evaluation of the Citizens' Assembly on the Inquiry of Long-Term Funding of Adult Social Care, Newcastle: Newcastle University, Available from: http://whatworksscotland.ac.uk/wp-content/uploads/2021/02/SPCJLongTermFundingAdultSocialCare.pdf [Accessed on 17 January 2022].

Emmerson, C. and Stockton, I. (2021) Outlook for the public finances, Book Chapter, Institute for Fiscal Studies Green Budget 2021, Available from: https://ifs.org.uk/publications/15692 [Accessed 17 January 2022].

European Commission, Directorate-General for Employment, Social Affairs and Inclusion (2021) Long-term care report: Trends, challenges and opportunities in an ageing society, Volume I, Publications Office, Available at https://data.europa.eu/doi/10.2767/677726. [Accessed 14 December 2021].

European Commission, Directorate-General for Employment, Social Affairs and Inclusion (2021a) Long-term care report: Trends, challenges and opportunities in an ageing society, Volume II, Country Profiles, Publications Office, Available from: https://data.europa.eu/doi/10.2767/183997/ [Accessed 14 December 2021].

European Social Network (2021) COVID-19 Impact on Europe's Social Services: Protecting the Most Vulnerable in Times of Crisis, Brussels: European Social Network.

Evans, J. (2003) The Independent Living Movement in the UK, Independent Living Institute, Available from: https://www.independentliving.org/docs6/evans2003.html [Accessed 17 January 2022].

Ewbank, L., Thompson, J., McKenna, H., Anandaciva, S. and Ward, D. (2021) NHS hospital bed numbers: Past, present, future, The King's Fund, Available from: https://www.kingsfund.org.uk/publications/nhs-hospital-bed-numbers [Accessed 17 January 2022].

Fernandez, J.L. and Forder, J. (2008) Consequences of local variations in social care on the performance of the acute health care sector, Applied Economics 40(12): 1503–18, DOI:10.1080/00036840600843939

Financial Times (2021) UK industrial strategy refresh ditched as ministers set out plan for growth, 9 February, Available at: https://www.ft.com/content/013ce682-09c8-4132-9a14-232f7e9f311a [Accessed 17 January 2022].

Financial Times (2021a) Rishi Sunak looks to insurers to help with social care costs, 10 September, Available from: https://www.ft.com/content/c45723f4-0554- 423e-9a82-8aa340148fc7 [Accessed 17 January 2022].

Fisher, R. (2019) The perils of short-termism: Civilisation's greatest threat, BBC, Available from: https://www.bbc.com/future/article/20190109-the-perils-of-short-termism-civilisations-greatest-threat [Accessed 15 December 2021].

Foot, M. (2009) Aneurin Bevan: A Biography, Vol 2, 1879–1945, London: Faber and Faber.

Forder, J. (2018) The impact and cost of adult social care: Marginal effects of changes in funding, Quality and Outcomes of Person Centred Care Research Unit Discussion Paper 2946, Available from: https://www.pssru.ac.uk/pub/5425.pdf [Accessed 6 December 2021].

Forder, J. and Fernandez, J.L. (2011b) What works abroad? Evaluating the funding of long-term care: International perspectives, Discussion Paper 2794, Kent: PSSRU.

Foster, D. (2021) Adult social care: Means-test parameters since 1997, London: House of Commons Library, Available from: http://researchbriefings.files.parliament.uk/documents/CBP-8005/CBP-8005.pdf [Accessed 10 December 2022].

Foster, D. (2022) Adult social care funding (England), no 7903, London: House of Commons Library.

Fox, A. (2018) A New Health and Social Care System: Escaping the Invisible Asylum, Bristol: Policy Press.

Garrett, H., Mackay, M., Nicol, S., Piddington, J. and Roys, M. (2021) Briefing paper: The cost of poor housing in England, Watford: Buildings Research Establishment, Available from: https://www.bre.co.uk/filelibrary/pdf/87741-Cost-of-Poor-Housing-Briefing-Paper-v3.pdf [Accessed 19 December 2021].

Goldin, I. (2021) Rescue: From Global Crisis to a Better World, London: Hodder & Stoughton.

Golding, N. (2020) Can Churchill rescue Dilnot? Local Government Chronicle, 16 October, Available from: https://www.lgcplus.com/politics/lgc-briefing/can-churchill-rescue-dilnot-16-10-2020/ [Accessed 17 January 2022].

Gori, C., Fernandez, J.L. and Wittenberg, R. (2016) Long-Term Care in OECD Countries, Bristol: Policy Press.

Gramsci, A. (1971) Selection from the Prison Notebooks of Antonio Gramsci (edited and translated by Quinton Hoare and Geoffrey Nowell Smith), London: Lawrence & Wishart.

Gratton, L. and Scott, A. (2016) The 100-Year Life: Living and Working in an Age of Longevity, London: Bloomsbury.

Green, D. (2020) Fixing the Care Crisis, London: Centre for Policy Studies.

Griffiths, R. (1988) Community Care: An Agenda for Action, London: HMSO.

Gustafsson, M. (2019) Mapping millennials' living standards, London: Resolution Foundation, Available from: https://www.resolutionfoundation.org/publications/mapping-millennials-living-standards/ [Accessed November 4 2021].

Ham, C. (2022) Governing the health and care system in England: Creating conditions for success, London: NHS Confederation.

Hansard (House of Lords Debates) (2020) 9 January, Vol 801, Col 372, Available from: https://hansard.parliament.uk/Lords/2020-01-09/debates/8D354643-AF8F-4906-A0F8-CC4A027D47AD/Queen%E2%80%99SSpeech?highlight=queen%27s%20speech%202020#main-content [Accessed 23 September 2021].

Hansard (House of Lords Debates) (2020a) 28 October, Vol 807 Col 226, Available from: https://hansard.parliament.uk/Lords/2020-10-28/debates/D9B0BFA4-0C47-46D1-B9C8-CE92CFFEFB9D/SocialCare [Accessed 17 January 2022].

Hansard (House of Lords Debates) (2022) Health and Care Bill Volume 818, 31 January, Col 739, Available from: https://hansard.parliament.uk/Lords/2022-01-31/debates/1F90F71B-0C16-451F-9D08-33CBFFDFBE15/HealthAndCareBill#contribution-52AEFC4C-2255-42C4-BB8E-CE4BF368A41A [Accessed 6 February 2022].

Harrisson, T. (1976) Living Through the Blitz, Middlesex: Penguin.

Hayashi, M. (2011) The care of older people in Japan: Myths and realities of family care, History & Policy, 3 June, Available from: www. historyandpolicy.org/index.php/policy-papers/papers/the-care-of-older-people-in-japan-myths-and-realities-of-family-care [Accessed 17 January 2022].

Health Foundation (2021) Last minute changes to social care reforms are a step in the wrong direction, Press Release, 18 November, Available from: https://www.health.org.uk/news-and-comment/ news/last-minute-changes-to-social-care-reforms-are-a-step-in-the-wrong-direction [Accessed 17 January 2022].

Health and Social Care and Housing, Communities and Local Government Committees (2018) Long-term funding of adult social care: First Joint report of the Health and Social Care and Housing, Communities and Local Government Committees of Session 2017–19 HC768, Available from: https://publications.parliament. uk/pa/cm201719/cmselect/cmcomloc/768/768.pdf [Accessed 17 January 2022].

Health and Social Care Committee (2020a) Oral evidence: Management of the coronavirus outbreak, HC 206, 9 June, Available from: https:// committees.parliament.uk/oralevidence/482/html [Accessed 4 January 2022].

Health and Social Care Committee (2020) Oral evidence: Social care – funding and workforce, HC 206, 23 June, Available from: https:// committees.parliament.uk/writtenevidence/10906/html [Accessed 17 January 2022].

Health and Social Care Committee (2021) Social care: funding and workforce, Third Report of Session 2019–21, HC 206, Available from: https://committees.parliament.uk/publications/3120/docume nts/29193/default/ [Accessed 11 January 2022].

Health and Social Care Committee (2021a) Oral evidence: Supporting those with dementia and their carers, HC 96, 18 May, Available from: https://committees.parliament.uk/oralevidence/2189/pdf/ [Accessed 17 January 2022].

Heaven, W. (2017) The Tory 'dementia tax' could backfire for Theresa May, The Spectator, 17 May, Available from: https://www.spectator. co.uk/article/the-tory-dementia-tax-could-backfire-for-theresa-may [Accessed 3 July 2021].

Hemmings, N. (2021) The adult social care workforce: Next in the Secretary of State's in-tray or last on the agenda? Nuffield Trust Comment, Available from: https://www.nuffieldtrust.org.uk/news-item/the-adult-social-care-workforce-next-in-the-secretary-of-state-s-in-tray-or-last-on-the-agenda [Accessed 17 January 2022].

Hennessy, P. (2006) Never Again: Britain 1945–51 London: Penguin.

Hennessy, P. (2022) A Duty of Care: Britain Before and After COVID, London, Allen Lane.

Henwood, M., Glasby, J., Mckay, S. and Needham, C. (2020) Self-funders: Still by-standers in the English social care market? Social Policy and Society 21(2): 227–41, Available from: https://doi.org/10.1017/S1474746420000603 [Accessed 18 November 2021].

Hirsch, D. (2006) Paying for long-term care: Moving forward, York: Rowntree Foundation, Available from: https://www.jrf.org.uk/report/paying-long-term-care-moving-forward [Accessed 17 January 2022].

HM Government (2007) Putting people first: A shared vision and commitment to the transformation of adult social care, Available from: https://webarchive.nationalarchives.gov.uk/ukgwa/2013010 4175839/http://www.dh.gov.uk/en/Publicationsandstatistics/Publi cations/PublicationsPolicyAndGuidance/DH_081118 [Accessed 17 January 2022].

HM Government (2009) The Big Care Debate: Report the Consultation, London: Central Office of Information.

HM Government (2009a) Shaping the future of care together Cm 7673, London: HMSO, Available from: https://assets.publishing. service.gov.uk/government/uploads/system/uploads/attachment_d ata/file/238551/7673.pdf [Accessed 17 January 2022].

HM Government (2010) Building the National Care Service, Cm 7854, London: HMSO, Available from: https://assets.publishing. service.gov.uk/government/uploads/system/uploads/attachment_d ata/file/238441/7854.pdf [Accessed 17 January 2022].

HM Government (2012) Caring for our future: Reforming care and support, Cm 8378, July, London: The Stationery Office.

HM Government (2017) Industrial Strategy Building a Britain fit for the future, Available from: https://assets.publishing.service.gov.uk/government/uploads/system/uploads/attachment_data/file/664563/industrial-strategy-white-paper-web-ready-version.pdf [Accessed 17 January 2022].

HM Government (2019) Boris Johnson's first speech as Prime Minister: 24 July, Available from: https://www.gov.uk/government/speeches/boris-johnsons-first-speech-as-prime-minister-24-july-2019 [Accessed 7 July 2019].

HM Government (2021) The Queen's Speech 2021, Available from: https://www.gov.uk/government/speeches/queens-speech-2021 [Accessed 14 December 2021].

HM Government (2021a) Build Back Better: Our plan for health social care, CP506, Available from: https://www.gov.uk/government/publications/build-back-better-our-plan-for-health-and-social-care/build-back-better-our-plan-for-health-and-social-care [Accessed 17 January 2022].

HM Revenue and Customs (2021) Direct effects of illustrative tax changes bulletin, updated June 2021, Available from: https://www.gov.uk/government/statistics/direct-effects-of-illustrative-tax-changes/direct-effects-of-illustrative-tax-changes-bulletin-june-2021 [Accessed 17 January 2022].

HM Treasury (2013) Budget 2013 HC1033.

HM Treasury (2021) Public expenditure statistical analyses 2021, CP 507, Table 10.1 Available from: https://assets.publishing.service.gov.uk/government/uploads/system/uploads/attachment_data/file/1003755/CCS207_CCS0621818186-001_PESA_ARA_2021_Web_Accessible.pdf [Accessed 19 December 2021].

Home Office (2021) Letter to the Migration Advisory Committee, 6 July, Available from: https://www.gov.uk/government/publications/commissioning-letter-to-the-mac-for-the-review-of-adult-social-care [Accessed 17 January 2022].

House of Commons Committee of Public Accounts (2018) NHS continuing healthcare funding, Thirteenth Report of Session 2017–19, HC455, London: House of Commons.

House of Commons (2018) Health and Social Care and Housing, Communities and Local Government Committees: Long-term funding of adult social care – First Joint Report of the Health and Social Care and Housing, Communities and Local Government Committees of Session 2017–19, HC768, Available from: https://publications.parliament.uk/pa/cm201719/cmselect/cmcomloc/768/768.pdf [Accessed 17 January 2022].

House of Commons Library (2019) Adult social care: The Government's ongoing policy review and anticipated Green Paper (England), Available from: https://commonslibrary.parliament.uk/research-briefings/cbp-8002/ [Accessed 17 January 2022].

House of Commons Library (2020) Briefing Paper CBP06128, NHS continuing healthcare in England, Available from: https://commons library.parliament.uk/research-briefings/sn06128/ [Accessed 17 January 2022].

House of Commons Library (2020a) Briefing Paper CBP07903, Adult social care funding (England), Available from: https://com monslibrary.parliament.uk/research-briefings/cbp-7903/ [Accessed 17 January 2022].

House of Commons Library (2021) Number 8001, Adult social care funding reform: Developments since July 2019 (England), Available from: https://commonslibrary.parliament.uk/research-briefings/cbp-8001/ [Accessed 17 January 2022].

House of Lords (2019) Social care funding: Time to end a national scandal, Economic Affairs Committee 7th Report of Session 2017–19, HL Paper 392, Available from: https://committees.par liament.uk/publications/19/documents/547/default/ [Accessed 13 August 2021].

Hudson, B. (2021) Clients, Consumers or Citizens? The Privatisation of Adult Social Care in England, Bristol: Policy Press.

Humphries, R. (2015) Paying for care: Back to square one? Blog post, The King's Fund, Available from: https://www.kingsfund.org.uk/blog/2015/07/paying-care-back-square-one [Accessed 17 January 2022].

Humphries, R. and Timmins, N. (2021) Stories from social care leadership: Progress amid pestilence and penury, London: The King's Fund, Available from: https://www.kingsfund.org.uk/publications/social-care-leadership (Accessed 20 August 2022).

Hunt, J. (2021) Our social care problem is now critical.so why the delay in fixing it? The Daily Mail, 11 May, Available from: https://www.dailymail.co.uk/debate/article-9568259/JEREMY-HUNT-social-care-problem-critical-delay-fixing-it.html [Accessed 17 January 2022].

Idriss, O., Allen, L. and Alderwick, H. (2020) Social care for adults aged 18–64, London: Health Foundation, Available from: https://doi.org/10.37829/HF-2020-P02) [Accessed 17 January 2022].

Ikegami, N. (2007) Rationale, design and sustainability of long-term care insurance in Japan: In retrospect, Social Policy and Society 6(3): 423–34, Available from: 10.1017/S1474746407003739 [Accessed 17 January 2022].

Ilinca, S. (2021) European care systems respond to the expectations and preferences of their citizens? Abstract for the international workshop on COVID-19 and long-term care systems: What have we learnt and what policies do we need to strengthen LTC systems? 6 and 7 December, Available from: https://ltcCOVID.org/2021/11/22/you-cant-always-get-what-you-want-can-european-care-syst ems-respond-to-the-expectations-and-preferences-of-their-citizens/ [Accessed 15 December 2021].

Ilot, O., Randall, J., Bleasdale, A. and Norris, E. (2016) Making policy stick: Tackling long-term challenges in government, London: Institute for Government, Available from: https://www.institu teforgovernment.org.uk/sites/default/files/publications/5225%20 IFG%20-%20Making%20Policy%20Stick%20WEB.pdf [Accessed 17 January 2022].

Institute for Government (2021) Tax policy in the real world: In conversation with former chancellors, Event, 9 March, Available from: https://www.instituteforgovernment.org.uk/events/tax-pol icy?utm_source=Newsletter&utm_medium=email&utm_campa ign=GH230512&utm_term=Tax&utm_content=Events&inf_cont act_key=0453a34045118777b2f44aa7f52b9b58680f8914173f9191b 1c0223e68310bb1 [Accessed 17 January 2022].

Institute for Government (2021a) Performance Tracker 2021: Assessing the cost of COVID in public services, Available from: https://www. instituteforgovernment.org.uk/sites/default/files/publications/perf ormance-tracker-2021.pdf [Accessed 18 December 2021].

Institute of Fiscal Studies (2021) Quoted in podcast 30 June, Behind the scenes at HM Treasury, Available from: https://ifs.org.uk/podcast/beh ind-the-scenes-at-HM-treasury [Accessed on 12 December 2021].

Institute of Fiscal Studies (2021a) An initial response to the Prime Minister's announcement: Health, social care and National Insurance, 7 September, Available from: https://ifs.org.uk/publications/15619 [Accessed 17 January 2022].

Involve and House of Commons (2018) Citizens' Assembly on Social Care: Recommendations for funding adult social care, London: Involve, Available from: https://www.involve.org.uk/resour ces/publications/project-reports/citizens-assembly-social-care-how-fund-social-care [Accessed 11 January 2022].

Ipsos Mori (2017) Economist/Ipsos Mori Issues Index, June, Available from: https://www.ipsos.com/sites/default/files/2017-06/issues-index-june-17-charts.pdf [Accessed 17 January 2022].

Ipsos Mori (2018) Understanding public attitudes to social care funding reform in England: Report prepared for the Health Foundation and the King's Fund, Available from: https://www.ipsos.com/sites/default/files/ct/publication/documents/2018-06/public-attitu des-social-care-funding-reform-ipsos-mori-2018.pdf [Accessed 12 January 2022].

Ipsos Mori (2021) Two in three support increasing National Insurance for social care reform or to reduce NHS backlog, Available from: https://www.ipsos.com/ipsos-mori/en-uk/two-three-supp ort-increasing-national-insurance-social-care-reform-or-reduce-nhs-backlog [Accessed 19 December 2021].

Ipsos Mori (2021a) Ipsos Issues Index: Public concern about COVID-19 continues to fall, Available from: https://www.ipsos.com/en-uk/ipsos-mori-issues-index-public-concern-about-COVID-19-contin ues-fall [Accessed 12 December 2021].

James, E., Mitchell, R. and Morgan, H. (2019) Social Work, Cats and Rocket Science: Stories of Making a Difference in Social Work with Adults, London: Jessica Kingsley.

Javid, S. (2021) Speech to Conservative Party Conference October 6, Available from: https://www.ukpol.co.uk/sajid-javid-2021-spe ech-to-conservative-party-conference/ [Accessed 16 January 2022].

Johnson, E.K. (2015) The business of care: The moral labour of care workers, Sociology of Health & Illness 37(1): 112–26, Available from https://doi.org/10.1111/1467-9566.12184 [Accessed 17 January 2022].

Jones, E. (2020) The Government must grasp the nettle of social care reform, blog post, Conservative Home, 14 October, Available from: https://www.conservativehome.com/platform/2020/10/ed-jones-the-government-must-grasp-the-nettle-of-social-care-reform.html [Accessed 17 January 2022].

Jones, N., O'Brien, M. and Ryan, T. (2018) Representation of future generations in United Kingdom policy-making, 102(September): 153–63, Available from: http://dx.doi.org/10.1016/j.futures.2018.01.007 [Accessed 17 January 2022].

Jones, R. (2020) A History of the Personal Social Services in England, Switzerland: Palgrave Macmillan.

King, A. and Crewe, I. (2013) The Blunders of our Governments, London: Oneworld Publications.

The King's Fund (2011) Paul Burstow on social care funding, video recording of breakfast event, Available from: https://www.kingsfund.org.uk/audio-video/paul-burstow-social-care-funding [Accessed 30 March 2022].

The King's Fund (2017) Paul Burstow: Putting people first, presentation at Digital Health and Care Conference, 11 July, Available from: https://www.kingsfund.org.uk/audio-video/paul-burstow-putting-people-first [Accessed December 4 2021].

The King's Fund (2019) What does improving population health really mean? Available from: https://www.kingsfund.org.uk/publications/what-does-improving-population-health-mean [Accessed 17 January 2022].

The King's Fund (2021) A short history of social care funding reform in England: 1997 to 2021, Available from: https://www.kingsfund.org.uk/audio-video/short-history-social-care-funding [Accessed 3 December 2021].

The King's Fund (2021a) The King's Fund responds to the social care cap change vote, media release, 23 November, Available from: https://www.kingsfund.org.uk/press/press-releases/social-care-cap-change-vote [Accessed 17 January 2022].

Kingston, A., Comas-Herrera, A. and Jagger, C. (2018a) Forecasting the care needs of the older population in England over the next 20 years: Estimates from the Population Ageing and Care Simulation (PACSim) modelling study, Lancet Public Health, Available from: http://dx.doi.org/10.1016/S2468-2667(18)30118-X [Accessed 17 January 2022].

Kingston, A., Robinson, L., Booth, H., Knapp, M. and Jagger, C. (2018) Projections of multi-morbidity in the older population in England to 2035: Estimates from the Population Ageing and Care Simulation (PACSim) model, Age and Ageing, Volume 47, Issue 3, May 2018, pp374–380, https://doi.org/10.1093/ageing/afx201 [Accessed 17 January 2022].

Kotecha, V. (2019) Plugging the leaks in the UK care home industry: Strategies for resolving the financial crisis in the residential and nursing home sector, Centre for Health and the Public Interest, Available from: https://chpi.org.uk/wp-content/uploads/2019/11/CHPI-PluggingTheLeaks-Nov19-FINAL.pdf [Accessed 14 December 2021].

Krznaric, R. (2020) The Good Ancestor: How to Think Long-Term in a Short-Term World, London: WH Allen.

LaingBuisson (1998) Care of Elderly People, Market Survey, Suffolk: LaingBuisson.

LaingBuisson (2021) Care Homes for Older People, UK Market Report, 31st edition, Suffolk: Laingbuisson.

Law Commission (2011) Adult social care, HC91 London: Stationery Office, Available from: https://s3-eu-west-2.amazonaws.com/lawcom-prod-storage-11jsxou24uy7q/uploads/2015/03/lc326_adult_social_care.pdf [Accessed 17 January 2022].

Laybourn-Langton, L., Quilter-Pinner, H. and Treloar, N. (2021) Making change: What works? London: Institute for Public Policy Research and Runnymede Trust, Available from: http://www.ippr.org/research/publications/making-change-what-works [Accessed 17 January 2022].

Learner, S. (2022) Government U-turn on mandatory COVID vaccine branded 'a joke' and 'too late' by care homes, 1 February, Available from: https://www.carehome.co.uk/news/article.cfm/id/1664289/u-turn-COVID-vaccine-care-homes [Accessed 11 February 2022].

Leeds Health and Care Academy (2021) Annual Report, Available from: https://leedshealthandcareacademy.org/news/leeds-health-and-care-academy-annual-report/ [Accessed 17 January 2022].

Lightfoot, W., Heaven, W. and Henson, J. (2019) 21st Century social care: What's wrong with social care and how we can fix it, London: Policy Exchange, Available from: https://policyexchange.org.uk/publication/21st-century-social-care/ [Accessed 17 January 2022].

Local Government Association (2016) Report: Learning disability services efficiency project, Available from: https://www.local.gov.uk/sites/default/files/documents/lga-learning-disability-s-d9a.pdf [Accessed 17 January 2022].

Local Government Association (2020) Seven principles for adult social care reform, Available from: https://local.gov.uk/adult-social-care-seven-principles-reform [Accessed 17 January 2022].

Local Government Association (2020a) 2020 Spending review: On the day briefing, Available from: https://www.local.gov.uk/sites/default/files/documents/Spending%20Review%202020%20On%20the%20Day%20Briefing_1.pdf [Accessed 17 January 2022].

Local Government Association (2021) Building back local, Available from: https://www.local.gov.uk/publications/build-back-local-building-back-better [Accessed 17 January 2022].

Local Government Association (2021a) Spending Review 2021 submission, Available from: https://www.local.gov.uk/publications/spending-review-2021-submission#priority-2-adult-social-care-and-public-health [Accessed 1st December 2021].

Local Government Association (2022) Councils could face budget blackhole amid growing concerns about underfunded adult social care reforms, Available from: https://www.local.gov.uk/about/news/councils-could-face-budget-blackhole-amid-growing-concerns-about-underfunded-adult [Accessed 25 February 2022].

Local Government and Social Care Ombudsman (2021) Annual review of adult social care complaints 2020–21, Available from: https://www.lgo.org.uk/assets/attach/6132/ASC-Review-2020-21-vF.pdf [Accessed 17 January 2022].

Mackenzie P (2021) Making democracy work, London: Demos, Available from: https://demos.co.uk/project/making-democracy-work/#:~:text=download-,report,-%F0%9F%96%A8 [Accessed 17 January 2022].

Martin, S., Longo, F. and Lomas, J. (2021) Causal impact of social care, public health and healthcare expenditure on mortality in England: Cross-sectional evidence for 2013/2014, BMJ, Open 2021, Available from: https://bmjopen.bmj.com/content/11/10/e046417 [Accessed 6th December 2021].

Mazzucato, M. (2018) The Value of Everything: Making and Taking in the Global Economy, London: Allen Lane.

Melley, J. and Holt, A. (2021) Care homes: Following the money trail, BBC News, Available from: https://www.bbc.co.uk/news/uk-59504 521 [Accessed 14 December 2021].

Miller, R., Glasby, J. and Dickinson, H. (2021) Integrated health and social care in England: Ten years on, International Journal of Integrated Care, 21(S2): 6, Available from: http://doi.org/10.5334/ijic.5666 [Accessed 17 January 2022].

Moore, C. (2019) Margaret Thatcher: The Authorised Biography, Volume Three: Herself Alone, London: Allen Lane.

Mosse, K. (2021) An Extra Pair of Hands: A Story of Caring, Ageing and Everyday Acts of Love, London: Wellcome Foundation.

Mueller, M., Bourke, E. and Morgan, D. (2020), Assessing the comparability of long-term care spending estimates under the Joint Health Accounts Questionnaire, Technical Report, Paris: OECD, Paris, Available from: https://www.oecd.org/health/health-systems/LTC-Spending-Estimates-under-the-Joint-Health-Accounts-Questionnaire.pdf [Accessed 17 January 2022].

Murray, R. (2021) Raising the levy: Will the new health and social care tax work? Blog post, The King's Fund, 9 September, Available from: https://www.kingsfund.org.uk/blog/2021/09/raising-levy-health-and-social-care-tax [Accessed 12 December 2021].

National Audit Office (NAO) (2017) Health and social care integration, HC1011, London: NAO, Available from: https://www.nao.org.uk/report/health-and-social-care-integration/ [Accessed 17 January 2022].

NAO (2018) The adult social care workforce in England, HC714, London: NAO, Available from: https://www.nao.org.uk/report/the-adult-social-care-workforce-in-england/ [Accessed 17 January 2022].

NAO (2020) Readying the NHS and adult social care in England for COVID-19, HC367, London: NAO, Available from: https://www.nao.org.uk/wp-content/uploads/2020/06/Readying-the-NHS-and-adult-social-care-in-England-for-COVID-19.pdf [Accessed 17 January 2022].

NAO (2021) The adult social care market in England, HC1244, London: NAO, Available from https://www.nao.org.uk/report/adult-social-care-markets/ [Accessed 17 January 2022].

NAO (2021a) Initial learning from the government's response to the COVID-19 pandemic, HC 66, London: NAO, Available from: https://www.nao.org.uk/wp-content/uploads/2021/05/Init ial-learning-from-the-governments-response-to-the-COVID-19-pandemic.pdf [Accessed 20 August 2021].

National Care Forum (2022) NCF Briefing: Recruiting from the Shortage Occupation List, Available from: https://www.nationalca reforum.org.uk/wp-content/uploads/2022/01/NCF-Briefing-Rec ruiting-from-the-Shortage-Occupation-List-v6.pdf [Accessed 14 February 2022].

National Disability Insurance Agency (2021) Understanding the NDIS, Available from: https://www.ndis.gov.au/understanding [Accessed 17 January 2022].

Naylor, C. and Wellings, D. (2019) A citizen-led approach to health and care: Lessons from the Wigan Deal, London: The King's Fund, Available from: https://www.kingsfund.org.uk/sites/default/files/ 2019-07/A%20citizen-led%20report%20final%20%2819.6.19%29. pdf [Accessed 10 December 2021].

NCVO (2021) National Civil Society Almanac 2021, Available from: https://beta.ncvo.org.uk/ncvo-publications/uk-civil-society-almanac-2021/ [Accessed 8 February 2022].

New York Times (2021) Every 8 seconds, an American turns 65. How do we care for everyone? – Ai-jen Poo on the economic potential of a public investment in child care, elder care and paid family leave, 7 December, Podcast Transcript, Available from: https://www.nytimes. com/2021/12/07/opinion/ezra-klein-podcast-ai-jen-poo.html?sho wTranscript=1 [Accessed January 4 2022].

NHS (2021) Introduction to care and support, NHS website, September 2021, Available from: https://www.nhs.uk/conditions/ social-care-and-support-guide/introduction-to-care-and-support/

NHS Digital (2019) Equalities and Classifications (EQ-CL) Framework, Available from: https://nhs-prod.global.ssl.fastly.net/binaries/cont ent/assets/website-assets/data-and-information/data-collections/soc ial-care-collections-2019/eq-cl_2019-20_framework.pdf [Accessed 17 December 2021].

NHS Digital (2020) Health and care of people with learning disabilities: Experimental statistics, 2018 to 2019, Available from: https://digital.nhs.uk/data-and-information/publications/statistical/health-and-care-of-people-with-learning-disabilities/experimental-statistics-2018-to-2019/condition-prevalence [Accessed 27 December 2021].

NHS Digital (2020a) Adult social care activity and finance report, England: 2019–20, Available from: https://digital.nhs.uk/data-and-information/publications/statistical/adult-social-care-activity-and-finance-report/2019-20 [Accessed 17 January 2022].

NHS Digital (2020b) Mid-year 2020–21 adult social care activity, Available from: https://digital.nhs.uk/data-and-information/publications/statistical/mi-mid-year-adult-social-care-activity/mid-year-2020-21 [Accessed 17 January 2022].

NHS Digital (2020c) Personal social services adult social care survey, England 2019–20, Available from: https://digital.nhs.uk/data-and-information/publications/statistical/personal-social-services-adult-social-care-survey/england-2019-20 [Accessed 17 January 2022].

NHS England (2014) Speech by Simon Stevens, 1 April, Available from: https://www.england.nhs.uk/2014/04/simon-stevens-speech/ [Accessed 17 January 2022].

NHS England (2020) Delayed transfers of care data 2019–20, Available from: https://www.england.nhs.uk/statistics/statistical-work-areas/delayed-transfers-of-care/delayed-transfers-of-care-data-2019-20/ [Accessed 29 December 2021].

NHS England (2020a) The framework for enhanced health in care homes: Version 2, NHS England and NHS Improvement, Available at https://www.england.nhs.uk/wp-content/uploads/2020/03/the-framework-for-enhanced-health-in-care-homes-v2-0.pdf [Accessed 11 November 2021].

NHS England (2021) NHS continuing healthcare and NHS-funded nursing care data: Q2 2021, Available from: https://www.england.nhs.uk/statistics/wp-content/uploads/sites/2/2021/11/CHC-and-FNC-Statistical-Release-Q2-2021-22_2JyeCy.pdf [Accessed 12 January 2022].

Nuffield Trust (2019) Why a 'risk pool' must underpin a social care system, Available from: https://www.nuffieldtrust.org.uk/files/2019-07/social-care-risk-pool-nuffield-trust.pdf [Accessed 22 January 2022].

Nuffield Trust (2021) Significant tweak to social care proposals will leave fewer protected from catastrophic costs, Press Release, 22 November, Available from: https://www.nuffieldtrust.org.uk/news-item/nuffield-trust-significant-tweak-to-social-care-propos als-will-leave-fewer-protected-from-catastrophic-cost [Accessed January 22 2022].

OECD (Organisation for Economic Cooperation & Development) (2011) Help wanted? Providing and paying for long-term care, Paris, OECD Publishing.

OECD (2017) Tackling wasteful spending in health, Paris: OECD Publishing, Available from: https://www.oecd.org/health/tackling-wasteful-spending-on-health-9789264266414-en.htm [Accessed 22 January 2022].

OECD (2017a) A system of health accounts 2011, revised edition, Available from: https://doi.org/10.1787/9789264270985-en [Accessed 22 January 2022].

OECD (2020) Focus on spending on long-term care, Available from: https://www.oecd.org/health/health-systems/Spending-on-long-term-care-Brief-November-2020.pdf [Accessed 22 January 2022].

OECD (2020a) Who cares? Attracting and retaining care workers for the elderly, OECD Health Policy Studies, Paris: OECD Publishing, Available from: https://doi.org/10.1787/92c0ef68-en [Accessed 22 January 2022].

OECD (2021) Health statistics (health expenditure and financing data), Available from: https://stats.oecd.org/Index.aspx?QueryId=109591 [Accessed 22 January 2022].

OECD (2021a) Pensions at a glance 2021: OECD and G20 Indicators, Paris: OECD Publishing, Available from: https://doi.org/10.1787/ca401ebd-en. [Accessed 6 February 2022].

Office for Budget Responsibility (2018) Fiscal sustainability report July 2018, London: HMSO, Available from: https://obr.uk/fsr/fis cal-sustainability-report-july-2018/ [Accessed 8 December 2021].

Office for National Statistics (ONS) (2015) English life tables, No. 17: 2010 to 2012, Available from: https://www.ons.gov.uk/peopl epopulationandcommunity/birthsdeathsandmarriages/lifeexpec tancies/bulletins/englishlifetablesno17/2015-09-01 [Accessed 27 December 2021].

ONS (2019) National population projections: 2018-based, Available from: https://www.ons.gov.uk/peoplepopulationandcommunity/ populationandmigration/populationprojections/bulletins/nationalpo pulationprojections/2018based#changing-age-structure [Accessed 28 December 2021].

ONS (2019a) Total wealth in Great Britain: April 2016 to March 2018, Available from: https://www.ons.gov.uk/peoplepopulationa ndcommunity/personalandhouseholdfinances/incomeandwealth/ bulletins/totalwealthingreatbritain/april2016tomarch2018 [Accessed 6 December 2021].

ONS (2020) Social capital in the UK: 2020, Available from: https:// www.ons.gov.uk/peoplepopulationandcommunity/wellbeing/bullet ins/socialcapitalintheuk/2020 [Accessed 16th December 2021].

ONS (2021) Care homes and estimating the self-funding population, England: 2019 to 2020, Available from: https://www.ons.gov.uk/ peoplepopulationandcommunity/healthandsocialcare/socialcare/ articles/carehomesandestimatingtheselffundingpopulationengland/ 2019to2020 [Accessed 6 January 2022].

ONS (2021a) Accessing adult social care in England, Available from: https://www.ons.gov.uk/peoplepopulationandcommunity/ healthandsocialcare/socialcare/methodologies/accessingadultsocialca reinengland#stage-1-getting-information-on-accessing-social-care- and-funding-support [Accessed 6 January 2022].

ONS (2021b) Coronavirus (COVID-19) related deaths by occupation, England and Wales: Deaths registered between 9 March and 28 December 2020, Available from: https://www.ons.gov.uk/peopl epopulationandcommunity/healthandsocialcare/causesofdeath/bullet ins/coronavirusCOVID19relateddeathsbyoccupationenglandandwa les/deathsregisteredbetween9marchand28december2020 [Accessed 4 January 2022].

ONS (2021c) Employee earnings in the UK: 2021, Available from: https://www.ons.gov.uk/employmentandlabourmarket/ peopleinwork/earningsandworkinghours/bulletins/annualsurve yofhoursandearnings/2021#employee-earnings-data [Accessed 7 December 2021].

ONS (2021d) Public sector finances, UK: November 2021, Available from: https://www.ons.gov.uk/economy/governmentpublicsectora ndtaxes/publicsectorfinance/bulletins/publicsectorfinances/latest [Accessed 21 December 2021].

ONS (2021e) Child and infant mortality in England and Wales: 2019, Available from: https://www.ons.gov.uk/peoplepop ulationandcommunity/birthsdeathsandmarriages/deaths/bullet ins/childhoodinfantandperinatalmortalityinenglandandwales/2019 [Accessed 27 December 2021].

ONS (2022) National population projections: 2020-based interim, Available from: https://www.ons.gov.uk/peoplepopulationandco mmunity/populationandmigration/populationprojections/bullet ins/nationalpopulationprojections/2020basedinterim[Accessed 14 February 2022].

Oliver, D., Foot, C. and Humphries, R. (2014) Making our health and care systems fit for an ageing population, London: The King's Fund, Available from: https://www.kingsfund.org.uk/publications/mak ing-our-health-and-care-systems-fit-ageing-population [Accessed 7th December 2021].

Oung, C. (2021) Through a glass darkly: The unseen crisis in home care, Online Comment, Nuffield Trust, Available from: https://www. nuffieldtrust.org.uk/news-item/through-a-glass-darkly-the-unseen-crisis-in-home-care [Accessed 1st December 2021].

Oung., C, Schlepper, L, and Curry, N. (2020) What steps are currently being taken to reform social care? Nuffield Trust Adult Social Care in the Four Countries of the UK Explainer Series, Available from: https://www.nuffieldtrust.org.uk/comment-series/adult-soc ial-care-in-the-four-countries-of-the-uk [Accessed on 4 July 2020].

Pearl, J. (2021) What time do you go to bed? Blog post, Think Local Act Personal website, Available from: https://www.thinklocalactp ersonal.org.uk/Blog/What-time-do-you-go-to-bed/ [Accessed 14 January 2022].

Peckham, S., Hudson, B., Hunter, D., Redgate, S. and White, G. (2019) Improving choices for care: A strategic research initiative on the implementation of the care act 2014, National Institute for Health Research, Available from: https://doi.org/10.13140/ RG.2.2.13037.13288 [Accessed 7 February 2022].

Peters, T. and Waterman, R. (1982) In Search of Excellence: Lessons from America's Best-Run Companies, New York: Harper & Row.

Phillips, D. and Simpson, P. (2019) Changes in councils' adult social care and overall service spending in England, 2009–10 to 2017–18, Institute of Fiscal Studies Briefing Note BN240, Available from: https://ifs.org.uk/publications/13066 [Accessed 15 December 2021].

Platt, D. (2007) The Status of Social Care: A Review, unpublished.

Productivity Commission, Government of Australia (2011) Disability care and support, Report no. 54: Overview and recommendations, Available from: https://www.pc.gov.au/inquiries/completed/disability-support/report/disability-support-overview-booklet.pdf [Accessed 14 December 2021].

Productivity Commission, Government of Australia (2011a) Caring for older Australians: Overview report, Available from: https://www.pc.gov.au/inquiries/completed/aged-care/report/aged-care-overview-booklet.pdf [Accessed 14 December 2021].

Productivity Commission, Government of Australia (2017) National Disability Insurance Scheme (NDIS) Costs: Study report overview, Available from: https://www.pc.gov.au/inquiries/completed/ndis-costs/report/ndis-costs-overview.pdf [Accessed 14 December 2021].

Ranci, C. and Pavolini, E. (2015) Not all that glitters is gold: Long-term care reforms in the last two decades in Europe, Journal of European Social Policy 25(3): 270–85.

Rawls, J. (1971) A Theory of Justice, Cambridge, MA: Belknap Press.

Raymond, A., Bazeer, N., Barclay, C., Krelle, H., Idriss, O., Tallack, C. and Kelly, E. (2021) Our ageing population: How ageing affects health and care need in England, London: Health Foundation, Available from: https://doi.org/10.37829/HF-2021-RC16 [Accessed 29 December 2021].

Redwood, J. (2012) Care For the elderly: The limitations of the Dilnot Proposals, London: Centre for Policy Studies, Available from: https://cps.org.uk/wp-content/uploads/2021/07/120814102855-CarefortheElderly.pdf [Accessed 8 February 2022].

Rees, M. (2011) Templeton Prize 2011: Full transcript of Martin Rees's acceptance speech, The Guardian, 6 April, Available from: https://www.theguardian.com/science/2011/apr/06/templeton-prize-2011-martin-rees-speech [Accessed 19 December 2021].

Report of the Committee on Local Authority and Allied Personal Social Services (1968) Cmnd 3703, London: Stationery Office.

Rigitano, E. (2018) COP24, the speech by 15-year-old climate activist Greta Thunberg everyone should listen to, Available from: https://www.lifegate.com/greta-thunberg-speech-cop24 [Accessed 12 November 2021].

Rivett, G. (2019) National Health Service history, Nuffield Trust, Available from: https://www.nuffieldtrust.org.uk/files/2019-11/nhs-history-book/58-67/powell-s-water-tower-speech.html [Accessed 4 October 2021].

Robertson, R., Gregory, S. and Jabbal, J. (2014) The social care and health systems of nine countries, London: The King's Fund, Available from: https://www.kingsfund.org.uk/sites/default/files/media/com mission-background-paper-social-care-health-system-other-countr ies.pdf [Accessed 14 October 2021].

Rocks, S., Boccarini, G., Charlesworth, A., Idriss, O., McConkey, R. and Rachet-Jacquet, L. (2021) Health and social care funding projections 2021, London: Health Foundation, Available from: https://www.health.org.uk/publications/health-and-social-care-funding-projections-2021 [Accessed 25 November 2021].

Rosling, H. (2014) How not to be ignorant about the world, TED Salon Berlin 2014, Available from: https://www.ted.com/talks/hans_and_ola_rosling_how_not_to_be_ignorant_about_the_world

Royal College of Occupational Therapists (2021) Principal occupational therapists in adult social care services in England: Roles and responsibilities, Available from: https://www.rcot.co.uk/sites/default/files/Principal%20Occupational%20Therapists%20in%20Ad ult%20Social%20Care%20Services.pdf [Accessed December 4 2021].

Royal College of Physicians (2022) Strength in numbers: Stronger workforce planning in the health and care bill, Available from: https://www.rcplondon.ac.uk/guidelines-policy/strength-numbers-stron ger-workforce-planning-health-and-care-bill [Accessed 4 April 2022].

Royal Commission into Aged Care Quality and Safety (2021) Final report, Available from: https://agedcare.royalcommission.gov.au/publications/final-report [Accessed 12 October 2021].

Ryan, S. (2020) Love, Learning Disabilities and Pockets of Brilliance: How Practitioners Can Make a Difference to the Lives of Children, Families and Adults, London: Jessica Kingsley.

Sanders, R. (2021) ESSS Outline: New models of care at home, Glasgow: Institute for Research and Innovation in Social Services (Iriss), Available from: https://www.iriss.org.uk/resources/outlines/new-models-care-home [Accessed 18 December 2021].

Schlepper, L. (2021) Capping the costs: What are the lessons from the German social care system? Blog post, Nuffield Trust, Available from: https://www.nuffieldtrust.org.uk/news-item/capping-the-costs-what-are-the-lessons-from-the-german-social-care-system [Accessed 1 December 2021].

Scottish Government (2021) Adult social care: Independent review, Edinburgh: Scottish Government, Available from: https://www.gov.scot/publications/independent-review-adult-social-care-scotland/ [Accessed 4 December 2021].

Scottish Government (2021a) Over £300 million new winter investment for health and care, Press Statement, 5 October, Available from: https://www.gov.scot/news/over-gbp-300-million-new-winter-investment-for-health-and-care/ [Accessed 4 February 2022].

Sen, A. (1999) Development as Freedom, Oxford: Oxford University Press.

Series, L. (2022) Deprivation of Liberty in the Shadows of the Institution, Bristol: Policy Press.

Shafik, M. (2021) What We Owe Each Other: A New Social Contract, London: Bodley Head.

Shannon, B. (2021) Identity, blog post, Rewriting Social Care website, 20 March, Available from: https://rewritingsocialcare.blog/2021/03/20/identity/ [Accessed June 4 2021].

Shrimpton, H., Cameron, D. and Skinner, G. (2017) Public perceptions of austerity, social care and personal data, Ipsos Mori, Available from: https://www.ipsos.com/en-uk/public-perceptions-austerity-social-care-and-personal-data [Accessed 4 January 2022].

Sibthorp, K. (2020) Commissioning: If you always do what you've always done, Social Care Innovation Network, 10 February, Available from: https://www.scie.org.uk/transforming-care/innovation/network/news-blogs/commissioning-always-do [Accessed 4 February 2022].

Skills for Care (2019) The state of the adult social care sector and workforce in England, September 2019, Leeds: Skills for Care, Available from: https://www.skillsforcare.org.uk/adult-social-care-workforce-data/Workforce-intelligence/documents/State-of-the-adult-social-care-sector/State-of-Report-2019.pdf [Accessed 27 December 2021].

Skills for Care (2021) The state of the adult social care sector and workforce in England, 2021, Leeds: Skills for Care, Available from: https://www.skillsforcare.org.uk/adult-social-care-workforce-data/Workforce-intelligence/publications/national-information/The-state-of-the-adult-social-care-sector-and-workforce-in-England.aspx [Accessed 4 January 2022].

Skills for Care (2021a) Individual employers and the personal assistant workforce, Available from: https://www.skillsforcare.org.uk/adult-social-care-workforce-data/Workforce-intelligence/documents/Individual-employers-and-the-PA-workforce/Individual-employers-and-the-PA-workforce.pdf [Accessed January 12 2022].

Skills for Care (2021b) Pay in the adult social care sector: Analysis of Adult Social Care Workforce Data Set (ASCWDS), February, Leeds: Skills for Care.

Skills for Care (2021c) Using the Care Friends app to support better recruitment and retention, blog, 19 October, Skills for Care, Available from: https://www.skillsforcare.org.uk/news-and-events/blogs/using-the-care-friends-app-to-support-better-recruitment-and-retention [Accessed 12 November 2021].

Skills for Care (and KD Network Analytics) (2021) The value of adult social care in England: Why it has never been more important to understand economic benefits of adult social care to individuals and society, Leeds: Skills for Care, Available from: https://www.skillsforcare.org.uk/adult-social-care-workforce-data/Workforce-intelligence/documents/The-value-of-adult-social-care-in-England-FINAL-report.pdf [Accessed 2 December 2021].

Skills for Care (2022) Vacancy information monthly tracking, Available from: https://www.skillsforcare.org.uk/adult-social-care-workforce-data/Workforce-intelligence/publications/Topics/COVID-19/Vacancy-information-monthly-tracking.aspx [Accessed 14 February 2022].

Smith, P., Phillips, D. and Simpson P. (2018) Adult social care funding: A local or national responsibility? Institute of Fiscal Studies, Available from: https://www.ifs.org.uk/publications/12857 [Accessed 8 February 2022].

Smith, R., Lloyd, L., Cameron, A., Johnson, E. and Willis, P. (2019) What is (adult) social care in England? Its origins and meaning, research, policy and planning, Research, Policy and Planning 33(2): 45–56. Available from: http://ssrg.org.uk/members/files/2018/02/1.-SMITH-et-al.pdf [Accessed 2 February 2022].

Smyth, C. (2021) Johnson blocking the tax rises needed to meet social care costs, The Times, 22 June, Available from: https://www.theti mes.co.uk/article/johnson-blocking-the-tax-rises-needed-to-meet-social-care-costs-s2fnn6xx5 [Accessed 2 February 2022].

Social Care Future (2019) Talking about a brighter social care future, Available from: https://socialcarefuture.files.wordpress.com/2019/10/ic-scf-report-2019-h-web-final-111119.pdf [Accessed 14 December 2021].

Social Care Institute for Excellence (2017) Asset-based places: A model for development, London: SCIE, Available from: https://www.scie.org.uk/files/future-of-care/asset-based-places/asset-based-places.pdf [Accessed 8 December 2021].

Social Care Institute for Excellence (2018) Social Care Institute for Excellence: Strengths-based approaches, Available from: https://www.scie.org.uk/strengths-based-approaches [Accessed 17 January 2022].

Social Care Institute for Excellence (2021) A place we can call home: A vision and a roadmap for providing more options for housing with care and support for older people, Commission on the Role of Housing in the Future of Care and Support, Available from: https://www.scie.org.uk/housing/role-of-housing/place-we-can-call-home [Accessed 18 December 2021].

Social Work England (2019) Professional standards, Available from: https://www.socialworkengland.org.uk/standards/professio nal-standards/ [Accessed 12 December 2021].

Sodha, S. (2021) Jeremy Hunt: this lockdown just isn't working quickly enough, The Guardian, 24 January, Available from: https://www.theguardian.com/world/2021/jan/24/jeremy-hunt-this-lockdown-just-isnt-working-fast-enough-COVID?CMP=Share_iOSApp_Ot her [Accessed 12 November 2021].

Statens Offentliga Utredningar (2021) Sub-report 2: Sweden during the pandemic, SOU 2021: 89, Available from: https://coronak ommissionen.com/publikationer/delbetankande-2/ [Accessed 8 December 2021].

Stein, J. (2021) Biden jobs plan seeks $400 billion to expand caretaking services as US faces surge in aging population, Washington Post, 2 April, Available from: https://www.washingtonpost.com/us-pol icy/2021/04/02/caregiving-elderly-white-house-infrastructure/ [Accessed 4 February 2022].

Sturrock, D. and Tallack, C. (2022) Does the cap fit? Analysing the government's proposed amendment to the English social care charging system, IFS Briefing Note BN399, London: Institute of Fiscal Studies and the Health Foundation.

Survation (2021) How to build public support to transform social care, Research Report, Available from: https://socialcarefuture.files. wordpress.com/2021/04/scf-final-research-report-how-to-build-public-support-to-transport-social-care-survation.pdf [Accessed 20 December 2021].

Sutcliffe, A. (2018) Don't forget the Mum Test! Blog post, Social Care Future, Available from: https://socialcarefuture.blog/2018/11/13/ dont-forget-the-mum-test/ [Accessed 16 December 2021].

Sutherland, S. (1999) With respect to old age: A report by the Royal Commission on Long-Term Care, Cmnd 4192, London: HMSO.

Swedish Government (2021) Sweden's elderly care system aims to help people live independent lives, Swedish Government, Available from: https://sweden.se/life/society/elderly-care-in-sweden [Accessed 18 August 2021].

Swinford, S. (2019) Exclusive: Theresa May warned plans for £100,000 cap care costs will require significant tax rises, The Telegraph, 22 February, Available from: https://www.telegraph.co.uk/politics/ 2019/02/22/exclusive-theresa-may-clashes-health-secretary-plans-100000/ [Accessed 2 February 2022].

Szebehely, M. and Meagher, G. (2018) Nordic eldercare: Weak universalism becoming weaker? Journal of European Social Policy 28(3): pp 294–308, Available from: 10.1177/0958928717735062 [Accessed 12 October 2021].

Tallack, C., Charlesworth, A., Kelly, E., McConkey, R. and Rocks, S. (2020) The bigger picture: Learning from two decades of change in NHS care in England, London: Health Foundation, Available from: https://doi.org/10.37829/HF-2020-RC10 [Accessed 6 January 2022].

Tallack, C., Shembavnekar, N., Boccarini, G., Rocks, S. and Finch, D. (2021) Spending Review 2021: what it means for health and social care, London: Health Foundation, Available from: https://www.health.org.uk/news-and-comment/charts-and-infographics/spending-review-2021-what-it-means-for-health-and-social-care [Accessed 18 December 2021].

Theobald, H. and Hampel, S. (2013) Radical institutional change and incremental transformation: Long-term care insurance in Germany, in Ranci, C. and Pavolini, E. (eds) Reforms in Long-Term Care Policies in Europe, Heidelberg, New York: Springer pp 117–38.

The White House (2021) Fact sheet: The American jobs plan, 31 March, Available from: https://www.whitehouse.gov/briefing-room/statements-releases/2021/03/31/fact-sheet-the-american-jobs-plan/ [Accessed 28 November 2021].

Think Local Act Personal (2018) Six innovations in social care, Available from: https://www.thinklocalactpersonal.org.uk/Latest/Six-innovati ons-in-social-care-/ [Accessed 14 December 2021].

Think Local Act Personal (2021) Direct payments: Working or not working? Available from: https://www.thinklocalactpersonal.org. uk/_assets/Resources/SDS/Direct-payments-Final.pdf [Accessed 16 December 2021].

Thom, J. (2021) Care Now, blog post, Tourettes Hero, 22 June, Available from: https://www.touretteshero.com/2021/06/22/care-now/ [Accessed 26 January 2022].

Timmins, N. (2012) Never again? The story of the Health and Social Care Act 2012, London: The King's Fund.

Timmins, N. (2017), The Five Giants: A Biography of the Welfare State, London: William Collins.

Timmins, N. (2021) The most expensive breakfast in history: Revisiting the Wanless review 20 years on, London: Health Foundation, Available from: https://health.org.uk/publications/reports/revisit ing-the-Wanless-review [Accessed 9 February 2022].

Timothy, N. (2017) Nick Timothy: Why I have resigned as the Prime Minister's advisor, Conservative Home website, 10 June, Available from: http://www.conservativehome.com/platform/2017/06/nick-timothy-why-i-have-resigned-as-the-prime-ministers-adviser.html [Accessed 14 May 2021].

Townsend, P. (1964) The Last Refuge: A survey of residential institutions and homes for the aged in England and Wales, London: Routledge & Kegan Paul.

UK Parliament (2018) Letter to Prime Minister, 23 March, Available from: https://www.parliament.uk/globalassets/documents/comm ons-committees/liaison/correspondence/Correspondence-with-the-Prime-Minister-re-parliamentary-commission-health-social-care-18-3-2018.pdf [Accessed 23 July 2021].

UK Parliament (2021) Elderly Social Care (Insurance) Bill, Available from: https://bills.parliament.uk/bills/2872/news [Accessed 4 October 2021].

United Nations (2007) Convention on the Rights of Persons with Disabilities, Available from: http://www.un.org/disabilities/docume nts/convention/convoptprot-e.pdf [Accessed 14 December 2021].

United Nations (2017) Convention on the rights of persons with disabilities: concluding observations on the initial report of the United Kingdom of Great Britain and Northern Ireland, Available from: https://docstore.ohchr.org/SelfServices/FilesHandler. ashx?enc=6QkG1d%2fPPRiCAqhKb7yhspCUnZhK1jU66fLQJyH IkqMIT3RDaLiqzhH8tVNxhro6S657eVNwuqlzu0xvsQUehREyY EQD%2bldQaLP31QDpRclYD9HugAGTgZ4s76Qfl5t8 [Accessed 14 December 2021].

United Nations (2019) 2018 Active ageing index analytical report, United Nations Economic Commission for Europe, Available from: https://unece.org/DAM/pau/age/Active_Ageing_Index/ ECE-WG-33.pdf [Accessed 8 December 2021].

United States Senate (1969) Senator Everett McKinley Dirksen dies, Available from: https://www.senate.gov/artandhistory/history/min ute/Senator_Everett_Mckinley_Dirksen_Dies.htm#:~:text=Caution ing%20that%20federal%20spending%20had,73%20on%20Septem ber%207%2C%201969 [Accessed 15 November 2021].

Wanless, D. (2006) Securing Good Care for Older People: Taking a Long-Term View, London: The King's Fund.

Warren, S. (2021) Making decisions about social care requires tough choices, blog post, The King's Fund, 31 March, Available from: https://www.kingsfund.org.uk/blog/2021/03/making-decisions-about-social-care-requires-tough-choices [Accessed 4 July 2021].

Watkin, B. (1974) Documents on Health and Social Services: 1834 to the Present Day, London: Methuen.

Waytowich, N. (2019) The Long Con and the Overton Window, Toronto Guardian, 27 May 27, Available from: https://torontoguardian.com/2019/05/long-con-overton-window/ [Accessed September 2021].

Webb, A. and Wistow, G. (1987) Social Work, Social Care and Social Planning: The Personal Social Services since Seebohm, London: Longman.

Wenzel, L., Bennett, L., Bottery, S., Murray, R. and Sahib, B. (2018) Approaches to social care funding: Social care funding options, Working Paper, London: Health Foundation, Available from: https://www.health.org.uk/publications/approaches-to-social-care-funding [Accessed 21 December 2021].

Which? (2021) Later life care: What is changing? 17 November, Available from: https://www.which.co.uk/reviews/later-life-care/article/which-later-life-care-what-is-changing-arrNx2J98TEe [Accessed 5 January 2022].

Willis, R., Evandrou, M., Pathak, P. and Khambhaita, P. (2015) Problems with measuring satisfaction with social care, Health and Social Care in the Community, Available from: https://eprints.soton.ac.uk/374519/1/Accepted%2520Manuscript%2520ASC%2520H%2526SCitC.pdf [Accessed 4 February 2022].

Wittenberg, R., Hu, B., and Hancock, R. (2018), Projections of demand and expenditure on adult social care 2015 to 2040, PSSRU Discussion Paper 2944, Available from: http://eprints.lse.ac.uk/88376/1/Wittenberg_Adult%20Social%20Care_Published.pdf [Accessed 28 December 2021].

World Health Organisation (2020) Strengthening the health system response to COVID-19: Preventing and managing the COVID-19 pandemic across long-term care services in the WHO European Region, Copenhagen: WHO Regional Office for Europe, Available from: https://apps.who.int/iris/bitstream/handle/10665/333067/WHO-EURO-2020-804-40539-54460-eng.pdf?sequence=1&isAllowed=y [Accessed 16 September 2022].

Index

Index

investment in home care 206
investment in long-term care 221
private insurance 155–6
universal service, social care 226–9
unpaid care 73, 127
female carers 168
improved support for 223
lack of financial support
for 168–9
new deal for 235–6
users *see* care users

V

voluntary private insurance 154–7

W

Wales
Future Generations
Commissioner 210
Well-being of Future Generations
Act (2015) 210
Wanless, Derek 92, 104
review (2002) 92, 93, 96, 97,
104, 107
Warren, Sally 108–9, 115
Watkin, B. 38
wealth
accumulation of 36–7
distribution 36

personal 35–6
wealth tax 245
welfare services 25
welfare state
creation of 4, 189, 249
origins of 21
well-being
economic and social 105, 222–4,
226, 228–9
emphasis on 50
financial 47–8
National Assistance Act (1948)
49
principle for local authorities 56
promotion of 47, 49, 50, 56, 148,
194, 200
White, Tom 39
Wigan Deal 236, 237
Willis et al. 86–7
Wilson, Harold 201–2
'With Respect to Old Age' (royal
commission) 91
workhouses 51–2

Y

York, Archbishop of 194

Z

zombie policy 154–7